Between Mind, Brain, and Managed Care

Between Mind, Brain, and Managed Care

THE NOW AND FUTURE WORLD

OF ACADEMIC PSYCHIATRY

EDITED BY

Roger E. Meyer, M.D.
Christopher J. McLaughlin

Association of Academic Health Centers

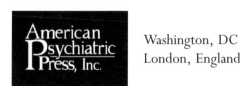

American Psychiatric Press, Inc.

Washington, DC
London, England

Copyright © 1998 American Psychiatric Press, Inc.

ALL RIGHTS RESERVED

Manufactured in the United States of America on acid-free paper

Supported by Grant # 95–33444 from the John D. and Catherine T. MacArthur Foundation

First Edition   01   00   99   98   4   3   2   1

American Psychiatric Press, Inc.
1400 K Street, N.W.
Washington, DC 20005
www.appi.org

Library of Congress Cataloging-in-Publication Data

Meyer, Roger E.
      Between mind, brain, and managed care : the now and future world
  of academic psychiatry / Roger E. Meyer, Christopher J. McLaughlin,
  — 1st ed.
        p. cm.
      Includes bibliographical references and index.
      ISBN 0-88048-815-8
      1. Psychiatry—Study and teaching—United States. 2. Managed
  mental health care—United States. 3. Psychiatry—Research—United
  States. 4. Academic medical centers—Effect of managed care on—
  United States. I. McLaughlin, Christopher J., 1966–   .
  II. Title.
      [DNLM: 1. Psychiatry—education—United States. 2. Psychiatry—
  trends—United States. 3. Managed Care Programs—United States.
  4. Education, Medical—United States. WM 18 M613b 1998]
  RC459.4.U6M49   1998
  616.89'0071'173—dc21   97-40588
                                                               CIP

British Library Cataloguing in Publication Data
A CIP record is available from the British Library.

To Sheila, Stephanie, and Jessica Meyer and Tobie and Ming-yuen Meyer-Fong—my family. Your support and understanding over many years continues to be the most important thing in my life.

Contents

Contributors

Thomas B. Horvath, M.D., F.R.A.C.P., is chief consultant for mental health for the U.S. Department of Veterans Affairs in Washington, D.C.

Christopher J. McLaughlin is program associate and manager of information technology at the Association of Academic Health Centers in Washington, D.C.

Roger E. Meyer, M.D., was a senior scholar in residence at the Association of Academic Health Centers in Washington, D.C., from 1995 to 1996. He is currently senior consultant on clinical research at the Association of American Medical Colleges.

Preface

Roger E. Meyer, M.D.

The idea for this book grew out of a sabbatical year (1992–1993) spent at the Center for Advanced Study in the Behavioral Sciences (CASBS) at Stanford University, where I had the opportunity to develop a study group on health care reform. My own interests concerned the impact of changes in the funding of clinical care on academic health centers and academic psychiatry. The latter issue had emerged in discussions among the members of the American Association of Chairmen of Departments of Psychiatry (AACDP), and at the Academic Psychiatry Consortium, which met yearly at CASBS. One can get a glimpse of the issues that I saw as emergent during that time in a paper that I wrote while at CASBS (Meyer 1993).

When I left George Washington University in 1995, I chanced to chat with my friend, Dr. Robert Rose, of the MacArthur Foundation. Bob and I had commenced our tenure as chairs in the same year. We had participated in the discussions at AACDP and CASBS regarding the future of academic psychiatry. He encouraged me to apply to the foundation to conduct a study on the impact of changes in the health care system on academic psychiatry. Drs. Roger Bulger and Marian Osterweis generously offered the Association of Academic Health Centers (AHC) as the host for the study, and provided me a research associate, Chris McLaughlin, as well as the able assistance of Serena Curry, Joan Durgin, Nancy Siegal, and Cynthia Spriggs. AHC was well-known to me as a dynamic organization that strives to bring together the educational lead-

ership for all health care professionals in the context of an organization
of Vice Presidents for Health or Medical Affairs. With AHC, I was able
to establish a distinguished advisory committee of leading academic psychiatrists, other academic physicians, advocates of managed behavioral
health care, and other mental health professionals.

The committee met on three occasions: at the outset of the project,
at the end of data collection, and to review a draft of the report. Ultimately, the views expressed in the book are my own and do not reflect
all of the collected wisdom of the members of the committee. I am
grateful that despite purposefully selected ideological differences on the
committee, there were no major objections to the general conclusions.
The committee was chaired by Dr. David Ramsey, who is president of
the University of Maryland–Baltimore and a distinguished leader in academic medicine. Dr. Ramsey was a constant supporter of the project—
and a wise diplomat in the process. I am deeply grateful to him and to
all of the members of the committee.

The other members of the advisory committee were Joseph Coyle,
M.D., Harvard Medical School; Mary Jane England, M.D., Washington
Business Group on Health; Saul Feldman, D.P.A., U.S. Behavioral
Health; Robin Jarrett, Ph.D., University of Texas Southwestern Medical
Center at Dallas; Robert Michels, M.D., Cornell University Medical
Center; Charles B. Nemeroff, M.D., Ph.D., Emory University School
of Medicine; Gregory Pawlson, M.D., The George Washington Univer-
sity; Robert M. Rose, M.D., The John D. and Catherine T. MacArthur
Foundation; James Shore, M.D., University of Colorado Health Sciences
Center; Helen L. Smits, M.D., Health Care Financing Administration;
and Gary Tucker, M.D., University of Washington.

This book is dedicated to the memory of Daniel X. Freedman, M.D.,
who served as long distance mentor for many leaders of academic psychiatry and research. Danny believed that the values of the academy
were the supreme values. His passion about the growth and survival of
academic psychiatry (and individual psychiatrists) made many of us call
him "the Godfather of academic psychiatry." As chair of psychiatry at
the University of Chicago, he early on established the importance of
research to the mission of our specialty. As editor of the *Archives of General
Psychiatry*, he presided over two decades of our science. As consultant
to many agencies of government, and in discussions with leaders in

Congress, he made others share his passion and commitment. Without Danny, many of the field's leaders feel relatively less well protected. He would not necessarily have embraced the recommendations of this volume—because, at his core, he believed that the world should make it possible for academic psychiatry to be academic psychiatry.

References

Meyer RE: The economics of survival for academic psychiatry. Acad Psychiatry 17:149–160, 1993

Foreword

Roger J. Bulger, M.D.

The publication of this book is a timely and important contribution to the growing literature and searching dialogue surrounding the impact of managed care on health services in general and on the educational and research efforts of our nation's academic (medical) health centers in particular. Typically, university-level academic health centers include at least two health professional schools (one of which is a medical school) and an associated hospital or health care delivery system. Even if the academic center has six or seven health professional schools, the largest financial player is almost always the medical school. We know that before the rapid emergence of managed care, subsidies from university hospitals and medical clinical faculties helped to support the costs of education and research in the medical school. These opportunities for legal cross-subsidization of the academic enterprise are rapidly disappearing, and it is just this impact that the authors have sought to explore within academic psychiatry. The analysis that has been produced has broad implications for psychiatry, for other core clinical disciplines, and for the entire academic health center. I believe that it may serve as a prototype for examining the impact of health care market forces on other academic specialties.

One test of the significance of a new policy analysis is the impression that it makes on knowledgeable observers. As a former dean, and as president of the Association of Academic Health Centers, I learned a number of things about psychiatry that I had not appreciated. Over the past 13 years, psychiatry has become one of the most research-intensive clinical disciplines within our medical schools. The range of research is extremely broad and includes new areas of investigation such as molecular and cellular research, clinical trials, psychiatric epidemiology, and services research. Despite massive upheaval in the public mental health sector in many states, the linkage between public sector and academic psychiatry is absolutely vital to both, and to the welfare of patients with chronic and severe mental illness as well. Public-sector support has also been essential to many academic psychiatry departments in the same way that surplus clinical income has assisted the procedure-based specialties to cover the unfunded or underfunded costs of education and research.

The undergraduate educational mission of psychiatry is one of the broadest of any discipline, with responsibility for courses in all 4 years of the curriculum. The new problem-based curricula are relying heavily on psychiatric faculty, as on their colleagues in the primary care disciplines. Psychiatry also resembles those disciplines in the problems that it has in managing its clinical programs within the usual structure of clinical practice of most academic health centers. Meyer and McLaughlin lay out these issues in great detail and offer some valuable suggestions to academic psychiatrists and leaders of clinical programs in our medical schools and teaching hospitals. Among a variety of recommendations, the authors urge departments of psychiatry to collaborate more closely with their colleagues in primary care disciplines and to develop new modes of practice that will serve to integrate mental and general health care. The traditional practice culture of psychiatry is being challenged, but the field needs to grasp the opportunities if it is to thrive and meet the needs of patients and families. All managed behavioral health care companies are not the same—and some of the leaders of this industry share a commitment to quality (as well as cost containment) with their colleagues in academic psychiatry.

Although the book does not directly address this issue, it has convinced me that psychiatry should not be merged with neurology—but that psychiatry does need to rediscover its humanistic vision of the biopsychosocial model within the context of new scientific discoveries and the new challenges of managed care. The problems facing psychiatric educators in this regard are closer to those facing primary care educators than to the issues facing academic neurology. I actually found myself excited by the prospects for the field, even as I was appalled by the excesses of marginalized care offered by some behavioral health care companies—and by the consequences of misguided public-sector policies that are obvious in the number of homeless mentally ill living on the streets of our great urban centers.

Dr. Roger Meyer, as principal author, brings an unusually broad range of credentials to this analysis. He is an internationally known academician with a distinguished research record at three different medical schools (Boston University, Harvard, and the University of Connecticut). Dr. Meyer served as department chair for 16 years at the University of Connecticut Medical School, where he helped establish the most research-intensive department in the school.[1] In addition to his service as chair, he was the principal investigator and scientific director of the NIH-funded Alcohol Research Center. Within the UConn Health Center, Dr. Meyer led the faculty practice plan for 5 years and served as executive dean of the medical school for 3 of those years. Roger's stature as a researcher was recognized by his peers in his election to the Presidency of the American College of Neuropsychopharmacology in 1992, and his leadership qualities as an academic psychiatrist were recognized in his election as president of the American Association of Chairmen of Departments of Psychiatry in 1990.

In 1992–1993, Dr. Meyer spent a sabbatical year as a fellow at the Center for Advanced Study in the Behavioral Sciences, where he organized an interdisciplinary study group on the impact of health care reform on academic health centers. In 1993 he had the opportunity to examine this issue up close as the vice president for health affairs and executive dean of the school of medicine and health sciences at George Washington University. There he had responsibility for a health maintenance organization (HMO), a faculty practice plan, a teaching hospital, and all of the educational and research programs of the medical school and the school of allied health sciences. During his tenure (1993–1995), the HMO membership grew by 32%, the medical center developed a significant cash surplus, and the faculty developed plans to reorganize

---

[1] Based on total grant support from the National Institutes of Health (NIH)/FTE faculty support from medical school.

the practice plan, to develop an infrastructure for research and graduate education in the biomedical and evaluation sciences, to start a school of public health, and to implement a significant international health effort. He elected to separate from George Washington University when leadership of the university decided to try to sell the hospital and the HMO.

Following his departure from George Washington, Dr. Meyer was able to secure funding for this project from the MacArthur Foundation. The Association of Academic Health Centers has been proud to host the grant. As president of the AHC, I would like to thank the MacArthur Foundation for its financial and moral support, without which this study would not have been possible. I am grateful to Dr. Roger Meyer for spending 15 months at AHC as Senior Scholar in Residence. He was a great stimulus for all of us and was a pleasure to work with. I would also like to thank Mr. Christopher McLaughlin, AHC program associate, for conducting the survey of psychiatry departments, analyzing the data collected, and serving as a coauthor of this book. Dr. Marian Osterweis, AHC executive vice president, and Ms. Serena Curry, AHC data coordinator, pitched in vigorously and productively in various essential aspects of this project, and I thank them as well. Deep and sincere thanks must be extended to the 10 distinguished members of the advisory committee (see preface). Their interest and active participation greatly affected the study design, and their responses to draft versions of the written report strengthened the final document.

Introduction

Roger E. Meyer, M.D.

It has now been more than 20 years since I became chair of the department of psychiatry at the University of Connecticut (UConn) School of Medicine. At that time, leadership was challenged by the imminent end of National Institute for Mental Health (NIMH) training grants for undergraduate and graduate medical education (including residency stipends), the need to identify internship slots following the restoration of the internship requirement, and the need to motivate faculty to carry out clinical activities and to bill through a faculty practice plan. Early in my tenure, it was also clear that the recruitment of psychiatry residency applicants was becoming a problem across the country, and the end of federal funding for community mental health centers thwarted our efforts to create an integrated public sector–academic psychiatry services program for the city of Hartford. Cassandras had warned of this end of academic psychiatry as we knew it.

Our department secured the first federally funded research center grant award at our medical school in 1978, established a base of academic psychiatrists and psychologists at the affiliated Veterans Administration (VA) hospital, implemented clinical revenue-generating strategies that kept the budget in the black, and shamelessly courted our own medical students in preclinical and clerkship rotations (so that more than 10% of the graduates of our medical school through the 1980s went into psychiatry). A base of UConn medical school graduates formed the core of each residency class during that decade; partially because of these accomplishments in psychiatric education, the director of our teaching programs went on to become chair at the University of Louisville in the early 1990s.[1]

While the strength of our program was diminished by the loss of key faculty at the affiliated VA hospital (and the end of our school's graduate medical education affiliations at the VA hospital in psychiatry, surgery, and radiology in 1989), the contemporaneous and long-hoped-for merger of our training programs with the Institute of Living promised marvelous resources for psychiatric education and clinical investigation. An affiliation with the addiction research programs at Yale, which also followed the end of the VA linkage, strengthened our research center in areas such as brain imaging, human genetics, and psychotherapy research.[2] While the research affiliation between UConn and Yale continues to thrive (see Chapter 4), the world of psychiatric practice and clinical education is vastly different today than that in 1989.

Rather than proving an asset, the Institute of Living's bed capacity and reputation for long-term psychotherapeutic care doomed its independence and diminished its value as an academic and research partner. As the psychiatry inpatient census at the university's hospital became increasingly dependent on Medicaid, the value of professional fee billings in psychiatry through the group practice plummeted as a consequence of the low fees paid by the government. The flat and relatively high dean's tax and the allocated costs of the faculty practice plan placed further pressure on psychiatry faculty to increase the percentage of time devoted to clinical revenue generation. By 1991–1992, the psychiatry faculty had reorganized itself into three academic interest clusters[3]—linking senior and junior clinician/teachers and researchers in an effort to preserve the academic mission for all in the context of our attention to the bottom line.

---

[1] Three other faculty who spent significant years at UConn also went on to become psychiatry chairs at other schools.

[2] Yale's research efforts were strengthened in alcoholism studies at the VA and at the Connecticut Mental Health Center and in a variety of services research areas in the addictions.

[3] The three clusters were built around the perceived research and clinical strengths in the department: psychological medicine/health psychology, adult psychiatric disorders, and addictions.

In spite of the strengths in research referred to by Dr. Roger Bulger in his foreword to this volume, the department's structural weaknesses in the 1990s involved its dependence on inpatient income at the university and the Institute of Living, the separate governance of the university and the department's largest clinical training sites at Hartford Hospital and the Institute of Living, the generic problems of psychiatric practice in a federated faculty practice plan, the absence of a strong academic–public sector relationship with the Connecticut Department of Mental Health or the VA, and a very limited research infrastructure for neuroscience in the medical school. The general relevance of these issues for academic psychiatry are highlighted throughout this book, but the silver-lined clouds of today are analogous to those in 1977. The Cassandras of this decade are right that academic psychiatry will never be the same, but the challenges facing today's generation of chairs also mean the opportunity to shape a different world for the field.

My own perspective on the issues has not been influenced only by my experiences as an academic psychiatrist, researcher, and clinician and as a department chair for 16 years. In 1987 I was asked by our dean at UConn to take over responsibility for the faculty practice plan, University Physicians. While the problems for psychiatry in the practice were apparent to me, it was also clear that the institutional responsibilities that I carried made it impossible to advocate for changes favorable to my own department. In 1989 I was appointed executive dean, with responsibilities for the practice plan and other issues of importance to the clinical departments (including the development of a General Clinical Research Center (GCRC), joint planning for clinical programs with hospital leadership, and strategic planning for shared programs in pediatrics and cardiothoracic surgery with our sister hospitals). The 3-year experience taught me about important differences in culture, governance, and values between academic institutions and excellent community hospitals; the challenge and importance of primary care services to the academic medical center; the obstacles and opportunities in operational and governance reform of faculty practice plans; and the broader issues of university governance, research administration, clinical education, and academic clinical practice. Academic psychiatry was not alone in its struggles and uncertainties; the quality of its survival would depend on the outcome for all of academic medicine.

In 1993 I left UConn to assume the position of vice president of medical affairs and executive dean[4] at George Washington (GW) University. The experience reinforced a view that academic health centers that could bring together the teaching hospital, practice plan, and medical school under a single governance structure were more likely to succeed in a competitive health care environment. The presence of a long-established HMO at GW highlighted other opportunities for academic health centers. But the experience also demonstrated the inherent financial conflicts between a relatively underendowed medical school and its similarly positioned parent university. Moreover, the inadequacy or inappropriateness of university systems of financial management, personnel, operations, and other administrative services weigh heavily on the teaching hospital and practice plan. The essential entrepreneurial culture of the health care environment is totally alien (if not threatening) to a university. In the absence of dedicated administrative systems, funding, and governance (which can also serve to protect the resources of the university from the risks of the medical marketplace), the clinical delivery system is at risk. As the pressures to downsize our academic capacity in medicine begin to accelerate over the next 5 to 10 years, these issues will need to be addressed by the trustees and leadership of our universities and academic medical centers. Institutions unable to adapt will not succeed.

The message to change or adapt in order to survive is one that also needs to be learned by academic psychiatry. After nearly 30 years as a faculty member at five institutions, I had not expected to learn much from this survey and case study process. I was pleasantly surprised. Despite real challenges to the viability of the academic mission, a number of departments are adapting well. The following conclusions emerged from the project, as well as from some antecedent biases. They are amplified in the chapters, especially Chapter 7.

The biopsychosocial model of psychiatric education and clinical care, which has been mostly displaced by descriptive psychiatry, needs to be

---

[4] As the reader can see, the title of executive dean was the same as that carried in a part-time role at UConn. Clearly the title had different meanings in the two institutions. At UConn, I reported to the dean of the medical school, whereas at George Washington I reported to the president of the university.

reclaimed. In its (relative) absence, the field has lost much of its relevance to the education of primary care physicians and medical students. Because these two areas of activity are critical to the future of academic psychiatry, we need to rediscover a biopsychosocial model for the twenty-first century.

Psychiatric education is more than residency training, and graduate medical education capacity needs to be downsized and made relevant to a managed care world. Continuing clinical education of the existing workforce is an opportunity for academic psychiatry departments—particularly if the effort can be linked to continuous quality improvement efforts of networks of allied mental health clinicians.

Linkages between academic and public-sector psychiatry are critical to the future of both.

Psychiatric research is at a very exciting stage. I believe that psychiatric research must be built on a solid base of clinical investigation tied to emerging concepts in brain and cognitive science. With the exception of the addictions, where the presence of homologous animal models of human behavior can serve as a link between molecular neurobiology and psychopathology, most of psychiatry is not yet ready for the insights of molecular biology (Meyer 1996). In a recent article, Andreasen (1997) highlights new studies that are coming closer to a linkage of psychiatric symptomatology and documented abnormalities of brain function.

Psychiatrists and other mental health professionals need to rediscover and update the multidisciplinary team of service delivery that they helped to pioneer more than 30 years ago. At this juncture, it requires some role definition, but psychiatric practice is not yet clinical neuroscience. In its care for persons with chronic illnesses, it is more like a combination of physiatry and primary care where treatment interventions may involve as much the art as the science of medicine.

Within academic health centers, psychiatric services will function best under distinct product line management that fosters collaboration among psychiatry departments and their colleagues in primary care practice. Collaborative care in these settings, and oversight of psychosocial services to patients with chronic illnesses (e.g., cancer), offers real opportunities for the future of the field.

If a psychiatry department is able to function within this type of setting, is able to access a strong public-sector or VA linkage, is well integrated into the research infrastructure of its parent medical center, and is supported for its broadly based undergraduate medical educational responsibilities, that department should be well positioned between mind, brain, and managed care.

References

Andreasen NC: Linking mind and brain in the study of mental illness: a project for a scientific psychopathology. Science 275:1586–1592, 1997
Meyer RE: Neuropsychopharmacology: are we ready for the paradigm shift? Neuropsychopharmacology 14:169–179, 1996

CHAPTER 1

Academic Psychiatry in an Uncertain Time

Roger E. Meyer, M.D., and Christopher J. McLaughlin

These are uncertain times for academic health centers (AHCs) (Iglehart 1994, 1995; Kassirer 1994). Over the past two decades, the AHCs have grown critically dependent on clinical income from tertiary and quaternary care to support the unfunded or underfunded costs of education, research, technology acquisition, uncompensated patient care, and community service. Although the number of medical students has remained constant since the late 1970s, there has been a huge growth in the number of faculty in clinical departments to service the patient care enterprise. In a world that valued the scientific basis of medical practice and freedom of patient choice of health care provider, the academic health center was in an enviable position. Knowledgeable consumers sought its specialists for care, industry valued and supported its clinical and basic science research mission, and government contributed substantial dollars to support its graduate medical education and research programs through payments based on direct costs, as well as formula payments for indirect costs.

Since the collapse of President Clinton's efforts at health care reform, the health care industry has been buffeted by market forces that have threatened the health care delivery system components of academic health centers. Managed care has favored primary care over specialty care, while preferring to limit the choice of health care provider to physicians and groups within their own networks. To compete for this activity, academic health centers have been forced to reduce their prices to approximate other providers in the community that do not have to shift "surplus" income to support education and research.

The opportunities for graduate training in some specialties have been undermined by the economic realities of excess capacity. The number of United States medical school graduates in some specialty training programs (e.g., anesthesiology) has plummeted in the past 5 years. The growth of the budget for the National Institutes of Health (NIH), while more favorable than for other parts of the federal budget, has not always kept up with health-related inflation, nor with the rich scientific opportunities across many fields of investigation. Assumptions about the beneficence of medical education and the production of biomedical scientists have been challenged by reports examining a perceived surplus of specialist clinicians (Billi et al. 1995; Wiener 1994) and scientists (Institute of Medicine 1990).

In the present climate, the balance of opinion and financial projections is more favorably disposed toward the education of generalist (primary care) physicians than the education of specialists and scientists. Within academic health centers, this shift in emphasis is having more of an impact on some specialties and subspecialties than others. The departmental structure (which historically formed the organizational, operational, and financial unit subserving undergraduate and graduate medical education, clinical activity, and research) is being challenged by the interdisciplinary organization of the curriculum, multidisciplinary centers of clinical and research excellence, and pressures to make clinical programs accountable to centralized planning and operational oversight. Some leaders of academic medicine have even questioned the continuing usefulness of the departmental structure in the medical school, apart from mentorship of junior faculty (R. Michels, personal communication, January 1997). At this juncture, there is a dynamic tension in many AHCs between the traditional role of academic departmental leadership and newly emergent models of clinical operational management (and separate structures of educational and research integration).

In this chapter I focus on the impact of changes in the academic health center and the health care environment on the mission of academic psychiatry. In this context, departments of psychiatry are experiencing some generic problems that are common across the academic health center, as well as some difficulties relatively unique to the specialty.

Within American medical schools and academic health centers, academic psychiatry departments are a relatively recent elaboration. To some extent, their development paralleled a period marked by the primacy of specialty training and the decline of general practice. As with specialty and subspecialty training in internal medicine and pediatrics, and the development of departments of family and community medicine, significant support for academic psychiatry came from the federal government and from foundations. The National Mental Health Act of 1946 established the National Institute of Mental Health (NIMH) as the primary funding source for the development of academic psychiatry and the training of psychiatrists and other mental health professionals. (Indeed, during the 1950s and 1960s, NIMH provided stipends to general practitioners anxious to be retooled as psychiatrists.) The teaching of psychiatry over the past 50 years in the United States has been characterized by a move from isolated practice and teaching in large state hospital facilities to practice patterns, teaching, and research that have brought the field closer to other areas of medicine. Unfortunately, as academic psychiatry has reached this point, academic health centers and medical schools are facing the broad array of financial pressures that threaten to undermine support for their academic mission.

I highlight how the present crisis in academic medicine, and the dramatic shift to managed care, is impacting on psychiatry departments across the country. Survey data from 48 departments of psychiatry[1]

---

[1] Separate survey instruments were sent to the psychiatry chairs and department administrators across 125 psychiatry departments. The questionnaires were completed by 48 of the 125 departments. Following repeated failed efforts to secure additional respondents from among the remaining department chairs or administrators, we conducted an independent one-page survey of faculty practice plan administrators relative to the operational characteristics of the practice plan for the department of psychiatry. Data from 25 practice plans, from institutions in which the department of psychiatry failed to respond to the survey, were gathered from the faxed responses of the administrative directors of the practice plans. These data were used to supplement data from the departments of psychiatry. In all, some date were obtained from 73 academic health centers.

(Table 1–1) and six selected case studies[2] will highlight how some departments have configured their efforts to meet the unique mission of academic psychiatry within health centers that differ in their emphasis on basic/clinical/health services research, tertiary/quaternary care, the

TABLE 1-1

Number of psychiatry departments, responding departments and practice plans, and case studies by region and ownership

Region	Ownership	Total number of departments	Departments responding	Practice plans responding with no department response	Case studies
West Coast	Public	8	3	2	0
	Private[a]	3	1	0	1
	Public/private	1	0	0	0
Mountain	Public	4	2	1	1
	Private	0	0	0	0
	Public/private				
Plains	Public	14	7	2	0
	Private	4	0	1	0
	Public/private	2	1	0	0
Midwest	Public	16	8	1	1
	Private	7	2	2	0
	Public/private	0	0	0	0
Southeast	Public	15	6	4	0
	Private	10	2	4	0
	Public/private	0	0	0	0
Mid-Atlantic	Public	12	5	3	1
	Private	8	4	1	1
	Public/private	0	0	0	0
Northeast	Public	7	2	2	0
	Private	14	5	2	1
	Public/private	0	0	0	0
Total		125	48	25	6

[a]Includes Charles R. Drew University of Medicine and Science.

[2] The five case studies from academic departments of psychiatry were selected from among departments that had provided very complete data about their finances

education of primary care versus specialist physicians, the education of other health (and mental health) care professionals, public service, and the clinical care of indigent patients. Important differences between public and private institutions (and between university-based and free-standing health science universities) also must be taken into account by departments of psychiatry and AHCs as they try to develop strategies to cope with the changing health care environment. There are important regional differences to consider in the context of the need for psychiatrists and other mental health professionals, as well as the "maturity" of the local market with respect to the impact of managed care on the organization and delivery of clinical services. For the most part, psychiatrists are concentrated in the Northeast corridor and California, and they are less visible in rural areas of the South and West.

Regional data describing the location of respondents versus all departments of psychiatry, their presence in public versus private schools, and the extent of managed care penetration in their local markets are presented in Figure 1–1[3] and Table 1–1. Across the United States, responses were received from 14 departments in private institutions, 33 departments in public institutions, and 1 public-private joint department (University of Nebraska–Creighton). Some additional operational and financial data were received from 25 practice plan administrators where there was no response from the psychiatry department. Of the responding departments and practice plans, more than half were located in markets where managed care penetration was at UHC stage II or III.[4]

---

and operations. Efforts were made to select cases that would reflect regional differences, as well as differences in mission (e.g., public or private university, research intensity, and degree of public-sector involvement). The brief case report from Sheppard and Enoch Pratt Health System was added to highlight potential innovative strategies.

[3] The extent of managed care penetration has been characterized as one of four stages (I, II, III, IV) according to the methodology developed by the University HealthSystem Consortium (UHC). This methodology classifies managed care markets as either being unstructured (stage I), having a loose framework of providers (II), having a consolidation of providers (III), or having a true managed competition environment with solid networks of providers (IV).

[4] Because the response sample was not random, and all respondents did not respond to all questions, the reader should be cautioned to avoid sweeping conclusions about the state of academic psychiatry as a whole. The report is best viewed as a

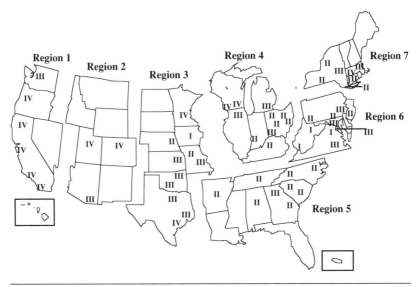

FIGURE 1-1. *Regional breakdown of managed care intensity based on the University Hospital Consortium stages criteria as applied to locations of the 48 respondent departments.*

In these times, the educational programs in academic psychiatry departments have been broadly affected by the degree of managed care penetration on the overall health center, by the specific consequences of managed behavioral health care on clinical practice and training, by changes in the medical school curriculum, and by the declining percentage of United States medical school graduates entering psychiatry. In general, the undergraduate educational requirements for psychiatry probably constitute one of its major points of influence within academic medicine. The National Board of Medical Examiners tests for competence in behavioral science and in psychiatry, and the Liaison Committee on Medical Education (LCME) requires medical schools to prepare all students in these areas of knowledge. In many medical schools, the psychiatry department carries one of the broadest areas of teaching responsibility across the 4-year curriculum. In a number of institutions,

reasonable overview of a segment of academic psychiatry in the United States in these rapidly changing times. The respondent departments provide a benchmark against which comparisons can be made. In this regard it is a relevant, though not a scientific, sample.

psychiatry faculty are playing a significant role in advancing educational programs based on problem-based learning.

In the next few years, changes in clinical practice and new developments in neuroscience will force a reexamination of the boundaries among the roles of psychiatrists, neurologists, primary care physicians, and other mental health professionals in ways that will impact on undergraduate medical education and residency training in each of these areas. At this juncture, departments of psychiatry differ in the degree to which they emphasize (if at all) basic, clinical, and health service research in their broad educational mission. Between 1984 and 1993, psychiatry moved from 10th place to 2nd place in NIH support among medical school departments (see Chapter 4), which has changed the emphasis and criteria for academic excellence (faculty appointments and promotions) in the specialty.

The Present and Future Profile of Academic Psychiatry Faculty

According to AAMC, there are approximately 6,400 full-time faculty in psychiatry departments across the 125 allopathic medical schools in the United States (Jonas et al. 1991). Approximately 57% of these individuals have M.D. degrees, which highlights the relatively high percentage of non-M.D. faculty serving the multiple educational and research objectives of academic psychiatry. Tables 1–2 and 1–3 break down the numbers of full-time faculty from respondent departments by rank, degree, and tenure status, with trends over time.[5] Unfortunately, it was impossible in this survey to compare trends in the 1990s with data from the previous decade. Because the earlier period was marked by a period of expansion in this field, one can surmise that from 1990 to 1995 there was a slowing in the growth of faculty lines for psychiatrists. Unexpectedly, the 20 departments that responded to this question projected significant increases in psychiatrist and nonpsychiatrist faculty across 8 of the 12 categories of rank and tenure status for the year 2000. In

[5] Only 20 departments offered data on their faculty profiles for 1990, 1995, and projected to the year 2000.

TABLE 1-2

Full-time psychiatric faculty in 20 responding departments
(1900, 1995, 2000)

Status	Title	1990 Count	1995 Count	2000 Estimate
Tenured	Assistant professor	4	2	4
	Associate professor	53	48	83
	Professor	119	122	142
	Total	176	172	229
Nontenured	Assistant professor	288	370	371
	Associate professor	111	133	148
	Professor	46	52	78
	Total	445	555	597
	Total psychiatric faculty	621	727	826

TABLE 1-3

Full-time nonpsychiatric faculty in 20 responding departments
(1900, 1995, 2000)

Status	Title	1990 Count	1995 Count	2000 Estimate
Tenured	Assistant professor	8	5	4
	Associate professor	30	29	48
	Professor	70	77	78
	Total	108	111	130
Nontenured	Assistant professor	128	167	156
	Associate professor	65	72	93
	Professor	28	30	54
	Total	221	269	303
	Total nonpsychiatric faculty	329	380	433

aggregate, these departments projected an increase of 14% in the total number of full-time psychiatrist faculty and a comparable increase in full-time nonpsychiatrist faculty. Given the likely impact of managed behavioral health care on academic psychiatry departments and threats to the financial base of academic health centers, these 5-year projections of faculty stabilization and growth may not be sustainable.

One can project that in the context of changes in the curriculum requiring more intensive mentoring by faculty and decreasing clinical income per patient hour, it is likely that full-time faculty will have less time for research not supported by external grants. They will also be working harder in their teaching and clinical activities. At a retreat in August 1995, members of the American Association of Chairmen of Departments of Psychiatry (AACDP) projected some "new roles for faculty," including "stand-up supervisors" to combine teaching and pa-tient care more efficiently, "primary care infiltrators" to become integral parts of the ambulatory primary care team, "mobile supervisors" and "retooled experts on managed care and briefer therapies in a variety of satellite clinics" to help the rest of the psychiatry faculty to work more effectively in managed care settings (Talbott et al. 1995). The draft document heralded a major change in the work environment for full-time faculty.

It is likely that some aspects of the teaching mission will require a substantial cadre of voluntary faculty who are themselves facing in-creased pressures on their clinical incomes. Table 1–4 describes the voluntary faculty pool available to the 20 respondent departments of psychiatry between 1985 and (projected to) 2000. Among these de-partments, the period from 1985 to 1990 was marked by an increase in the number of voluntary faculty across most ranks. For the most part, this trend continued through 1995, but a modest decrease in all ranks of voluntary faculty is projected to the year 2000 across these depart-ments. Nine of the departments are currently reimbursing voluntary faculty for their teaching efforts. Four of them do not expect to continue this practice, while three of the departments that do not now compen-sate voluntary faculty for teaching expect to be obliged to pay them for their efforts within the next 5 years.

TABLE 1-4

Volunteer faculty in 20 responding departments
(1900, 1995, 2000)

Discipline	Title	1990 Count	1995 Count	2000 Estimate
Psychiatry	Assistant professor	895	955	849
	Associate professor	297	302	288
	Professor	131	154	160
	Total	1,323	1,411	1,297
Other	Assistant professor	362	430	406
	Associate professor	116	140	136
	Professor	45	65	62
	Total	523	635	604
	Total volunteer faculty	1,846	2,046	1,901

Changes in Sources of Support of Psychiatry Faculty Salaries

In the past 15 years, the traditional and more recent sources of support of psychiatry faculty salaries have either declined significantly or disappeared. Until the early 1980s, training grants for undergraduate and graduate medical education in psychiatry were widely available from NIMH. The grants included support for faculty teaching time and stipends for residents' salaries. Career Teacher Awards were available from all three Alcohol, Drug Abuse and Mental Health Administration (ADAMHA) institutes, enabling young faculty to start academic careers in their areas of interest. With the ready availability of federal support in the 1960s and 1970s, most psychiatry departments did not have to compete with other medical school departments for resources from the school or principal teaching hospital. In a number of states, the public sector provided considerable support for academic psychiatry, and academic excellence was associated with sites involved in state-funded mental health centers and research institutes.

The public sector was substantially enhanced (from the mid-1960s through the late 1970s) by federal funding of community mental health centers. This program seemed to offer expanded cooperation between academic and public-sector psychiatry (even as it contributed to the relative isolation of psychiatry faculty from their colleagues in other academic departments). When federal funding for community mental health centers was curtailed by the shift to block grants to the states in the early 1980s, and state support failed to honor the original commitment to these programs beyond the early matching period, a number of departments were compromised by a precipitous decline in support for public-sector-supported faculty salaries and residency stipends.[6] Academic departments turned to income from professional fee billing, as well as enhanced research efforts, in response to new scientific opportunities and strengthened funding of research by the former ADAMHA institutes.

The most reliable source of clinical income during the mid-1980s came from professional fee billing on inpatient psychiatry units in teaching (general) hospitals and freestanding private psychiatric hospitals. Alleged abuses in the for-profit psychiatric hospital industry led to the rapid expansion of managed behavioral health care companies designed to reduce the use of inpatient facilities and limit access to extended outpatient care. Managed behavioral health care carveouts have had greater penetration across more markets than any other such disease-specific efforts (Oss 1994). Although cost-savings estimates are controversial (and definitions of degrees of managed care are variable), it appears that the percentage of health care spending devoted to mental health has declined substantially in the most intensively managed care environments. This decline suggests that managed behavioral health care has had a greater relative impact on payments to providers than managed care has had on health care expenditures in general (Frank and McGuire 1995).[7]

Because of the requirements of some of the managed behavioral health companies, academic departments of psychiatry may be excluded from participation in these contracts because of the costs of inpatient

---

[6] As described in the case reports from Maryland, Colorado, Dartmouth, and Louisville, public sector–academic partnerships continue to play a vital role for some academic departments.

[7] Indeed, this prevalence may indicate that health care rationing involves rationing of care to patients with mental and addictive disorders to a disproportionate degree. This issue is mentioned in Chapter 2 in reference to capitation rates that are too low to support appropriate levels of care for persons with chronic mental illness.

bed care in the principal teaching hospital, the involvement of residents in providing care, and/or a preference to use master's-prepared therapists (in the community) instead of doctoral-level psychiatrists and psychologists for ongoing care.

Exclusion from managed care contracts, when coupled with a decline in the capacity of the public mental health care systems of a number of states, has resulted in a growing percentage of uninsured or Medicaid patients in the inpatient psychiatric beds of a number of AHCs. The value of inpatient attending fees on these units has declined because of escalating bad debts and allowances. In some states, there is a major effort under way to "privatize" Medicaid under capitated arrangements. The for-profit managed behavioral health industry has begun to move vigorously in this sector. It is likely that the discounted fees for services under these new arrangements will be more unfavorable for the providers than those under the traditional Medicaid system. Parenthetically, although a number of academic health centers have been able to negotiate discounted fee-for-service or capitated arrangements with health maintenance organizations (HMOs) under the privatized Medicaid programs (and possibly for non-Medicaid populations), some AHCs have felt obliged to exclude the academic psychiatry department from the contracts because behavioral health services have been carved out through one of the behavioral health companies. This issue is highlighted in some of the case reports in this book.

The bottom line is that a number of academic psychiatry departments are caught between the proverbial rock and a hard place. Where services to addicted and mentally ill patients have not been eliminated but are covered under HMO contracts, primary care physicians serve as gatekeepers, and referrals to psychiatry are discouraged even within academic practice organizations. Where behavioral health carveouts have been implemented for patients under HMO and traditional fee-for-service health care, companies have been offering extremely low, discounted fee-for-service rates that diminish the potential role of full-time doctoral-level faculty in the ongoing care of patients or simply exclude the academic psychiatry department in general.

The times call for innovative approaches to patient care that are compatible with an academic mission. The case examples from Colorado, Dartmouth, and the Sheppard and Enoch Pratt Health System highlight the opportunities. The case example from Stanford focuses on the difficulties. Given the tremendous economic pressures facing academic psychiatry departments, it is surprising that more of the respondent departments have not experienced a serious deficit or downsizing of faculty and program.[8]

The Current Financial Health of Academic Psychiatry

An attempt has been made to secure data on trends in sources and uses of funds by departments of psychiatry since 1990. Given that current financial data were offered by only 33 departments, and trends in at least 20 departments across most categories were available only between 1992–1993 and 1994–1995, one should be extremely cautious about generalizing the financial health of academic psychiatry as a whole from this material. It is possible that the departments with some of the most financially favorable information responded to this inquiry, whereas departments in financial difficulty did not wish their situation to be known.

Despite the limitations in the database, it is of interest that a significant majority of the 33 respondent departments continued to experience increased income across all categories through 1994–1995. Also relevant is that although 50% of the 20 reporting departments had an increase in clinical service income in 1992–1993, 78% of these departments reported an increase in clinical income during 1994–1995 (despite the presumed impact of managed care). Does the apparent improvement in clinical service income across these departments of psychiatry between 1993 and 1995 reflect the impact of changes made to improve their performance under managed care? A longer-term perspective, as well as data from more departments, would be needed to

---

[8] Twenty-seven departments responded to the query "Did your department experience a shortfall in the past five years?" Fifteen departments (55.6%) responded in the affirmative. It is unclear whether this figure is more than, less than, or equal to the percentage of academic departments in deficit in other clinical disciplines at the same schools. It is also unclear whether this percentage is characteristic of all academic psychiatry departments in the United States.

determine whether academic psychiatry departments are in fact managing to cope with managed care.

Success was not clearly related to whether the department was at a public, private, or freestanding health sciences university, nor was it related to the intensity of managed care penetration in the geographic area. The case examples and additional solicited responses from some departments with impressive clinical financial data describe a diversity of strategies that are more instructive than the survey data themselves.

It is of interest that professional fee income (which would be most affected by managed behavioral health contracts) actually accounts for a relatively minor portion of total departmental income across most of the 33 departments (Figure 1–2). Of these 33 departments, 26 received less than 50% of their income from these billings during the last reporting year (1994–1995), whereas 18 departments received less than 30% of their income from this source. A significant majority of the respondent departments reported increased grants or contracts income

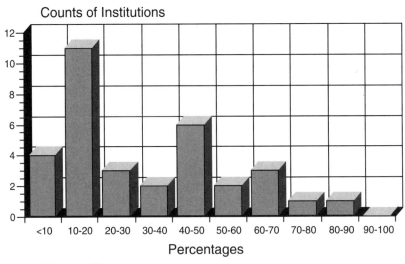

Institutions: 33
Average: 32.18
Std. Dev: 22.48
Maximum: 81.17
Minimum: 1.65

FIGURE 1-2. *Clinical income as percentage of total income.*

during 1994–1995.[9] The relatively large annual swings (increases and decreases) reflect the potential vulnerability of this category of funding to academic psychiatry. The average increase in grants or contracts income for 1994–1995 was 30.5% (SD 50.96%), while the average decrease was 22.2% (SD 12%). In the absence of some other substantial surplus in the budget that can offset the potential year-to-year losses in research support, it will be difficult for departments to maintain their research infrastructure from grants alone. In this regard, research grants to psychiatry departments are like research grants to AHCs in general. The challenge to academic health centers will be to develop mechanisms to fund their essential research infrastructure, which now includes the broad portfolio of psychiatric research.

One final point on the revenue side: approximately one-third of the respondent departments experienced a decrease in support from their medical schools for each of the 3 years for which we have trend data. In the context of managed behavioral health care exclusions that may impact negatively on departmental clinical income, and in the face of uncertainties in ongoing grant support, general fund support becomes ever more critical to the academic mission. These funds, plus a variety of revenue-generating opportunities for psychiatry within the AHC and in the public sector, represent critical support for the educational mission.

On the expense side, the number of respondent departments that reported paying increased professional salaries for 1994–1995 dropped substantially compared with the number of departments that reported paying increases in 1992–1993 and 1993–1994. This decrease appeared to be the most dramatic change in expenses among the departments reporting annual trend data. Again, it is too soon to tell whether and where departments will be pushing a cost-reduction strategy, although some of the case examples highlight what is happening at the local level in relation to cost reductions (e.g., in travel and administrative support staff).

Table 1–5 lists the types of consequences faced by the 15 responding departments that had experienced shortfalls in the previous 5 years. In two cases, the shortfall resulted in the chairperson stepping down. In

---

[9] Of the 33 respondent departments, 7 did not report any income in this category.

TABLE 1-5

Consequences of deficits in 15 responding departments

1. New department chair appointed and all psychiatric inpatient beds at the medical center closed.
2. Postdoctoral psychology positions reduced. Productivity process initiated to evaluate full-time faculty members on a monthly basis.
3. Faculty and staff downsized, salaries constrained, units consolidated, beds reduced, costs reduced, and cost-efficiencies implemented.
4. Practice revenues tapped to cover deficit.
5. Support positions eliminated, provider staff laid off, recruitment delayed, supply and other expense budgets cut, and department funds tapped to cover deficit.
6. Travel and perks limited.
7. Deficit this year will be covered from reserves. If revenue does not increase in next year, expenses will be decreased by lowering salaries.
8. Leadership replaced, faculty income decreased, and more focus placed on service delivery to provide income.
9. Shortfall intentional due to a major growth phase. Budget has been balanced for last 1.5 years.
10. Department selectively downsized, focused on priorities, and increased efficiency over a 3- to 4-year period. Resulted in some initial morale problems, but everyone is now working harder and the quality of the programs has been maintained.
11. Supervision of expenditures by the dean tightened, hiring frozen for support staff, and travel benefits for faculty eliminated.
12. Receivership assumed by campus health services foundation and financial oversight committee appointed; however, daily operations have been unaffected and salaries have not been reduced.
13. Shortfall represented less than 10% of reserves, and consequences have been minimal up to this point (e.g., no faculty bonuses).
14. Deficit resulted in staff reductions for nonfaculty positions, elimination of perks, and increased clinical workload for faculty.
15. Additional faculty not hired and budget not increased for program development.

at least eight cases, there were mandated staff reductions and other efforts to reduce costs. Although 20 of the 27 departments responding to the question of a deficit indicated that their deans distribute dollars from the dean's tax to departments that cannot meet budget from other sources, it is clear that this option has not been employed as a long-term strategy. Departments are obliged to meet budget, and they are usually expected to "pay back" the dean's fund for dollars "borrowed" to cover a shortfall.

The Structural Problems Facing Academic Psychiatry Within the AHC

Within the AHC, academic psychiatry programs share certain characteristics with departments of pediatrics and certain subspecialties of internal medicine. These departments carry a disproportionate share of the teaching and are least able to support teaching and research through clinical income. They also often must bear the full burden of practice costs (e.g., clinical practice space and physician extenders). In contrast, some departments with fewer educational responsibilities (e.g., radiology, anesthesiology, and surgical subspecialties) have been able to generate surplus clinical income while carrying few burdens associated with the cost of their practice environment (e.g., the costs of space and physician extenders in the operating room and radiology suite). Indeed, in many AHCs these department heads have successfully argued that they must be able to pay full-time faculty clinicians salaries comparable to what they would earn in the private sector. In AHCs without a multispecialty group practice mentality, they have argued against group practice modes of governance—and they generally have believed that funds cannot be diverted from competitive subspecialist salaries to support the costs of research and education in the department or the medical school.[10] Over the past 30 years, as AHCs emphasized the high-tech and subspecialty requirements of tertiary and quaternary care under the fee-for-service system, they became addicted to this source of funding and were not inclined to deny requests for additional subspecialist faculty and technology, even if they added little to the educational mission.

While the relative reimbursement patterns for physicians and surgeons in AHCs have not differed from those of the private sector, the academic health centers' reliance on clinical dollars to support some unfunded costs of research and education has fueled the dependence on

---

[10] In most communities, this argument has had real validity in fee-for-service medicine. Subspecialists would relocate to competitor hospitals if they felt disadvantaged at the AHC. However, as described in the case report from Dartmouth (Lahey-Hitchcock Clinic), this attitude among surgical subspecialists does not appear to occur in a true multispecialty group. A comparison of the clinical practice culture (e.g., salaries of surgical subspecialists versus primary care physicians) at the Dartmouth Hitchcock Medical Center with that at the University of Vermont would be instructive.

subspecialists. As AHCs confront the new world of managed health care, they are being forced to face the consequences of their traditional clinical program and management structures. The models of clinical operations, cost allocations, and fee structures that served the fee-for-service practice management needs of the subspecialists are less functional in a cost-sensitive managed care environment—especially for primary care providers. The one-stop-shopping opportunity of faculty practice is undermined by the traditional departmental or federated organizational structure of the clinical operations. Moreover, it is difficult to sustain the rates of reimbursement to some of the academic subspecialists while attempting to cut costs from the system as a whole.[11]

In addition to bearing the costs of the academic mission, psychiatry departments face some of the same types of structural problems that have historically plagued primary care divisions and departments within the usual practice environment of the AHC. However, in the new world of managed care, primary care programs have become critical to the future of academic medicine, creating the need for special subsidies in some settings. Psychiatry departments do not bring the same relative value in the context of potential referrals to the tertiary- or quaternary-care system.

Within faculty practice plans, the overhead charges for the administration of the plan may be anticompetitive in the managed care marketplace. In systems that charge business expenses to departments on the basis of number of transactions rather than as a percentage of charges, psychiatry (like primary care) pays a disproportionate share of the operating costs of the practice. Where the costs of malpractice insurance are distributed across departments to shield some departments from the confiscatory rates associated with the specialty, academic psychiatry is taxed well above the rate that its competition in the community is paying. In schools with a flat rather than a graduated dean's tax, higher-

---

[11] Some institutions are experimenting with product-line management (e.g., heart or cancer programs) that facilitate capitation strategies by "bundling" professional and hospital fees across all specialties and levels of care. In the best of worlds, the higher-paid subspecialists can develop a stake in the development of multidisciplinary centers of clinical, research, and educational excellence that can serve to strengthen their reputations and referrals.

earning specialties have distinct financial advantages over primary care disciplines and psychiatry.

Overall, it is our impression that the "average" department of psychiatry collects approximately 50% of billed charges for professional services. If the department is serving a large Medicaid or medically indigent population, those percentages are substantially less than 50% because of bad debts and allowances.[12] In a reasonably intensive managed care environment such as Washington, D.C., the usual and customary fee for 50 minutes of psychotherapy in a psychiatrist's office is $150. Managed behavioral health care companies will pay $65 for this service. If the service is delivered in an academic department of psychiatry that receives 50% of billed charges on insured patients, the department will actually collect $32.50 per hour of faculty time. In a typical academic environment, a psychiatrist may bill for 30 hours of patient care per week for 48 weeks per year. In a fully managed behavioral health care or discounted fee-for-service practice, that psychiatrist's clinical activity will bring in $46,800 per year. These numbers highlight the financial dimensions of the problem.

Until recently, professional fee billing on inpatient psychiatric services produced a modest profit, enabling departments to balance their books relative to overall clinical activity. With case-based rates for inpatient care, this balancing act is no longer possible in many locations. The example also highlights the financial burdens placed on academic psychiatry departments within the tax structure of most faculty practice plans and medical schools. The data highlight the rationale behind strategies that have emphasized public-sector contracts (Maryland, Colorado, Louisville, and Dartmouth) and efforts to create affiliated networks of clinicians (see Chapter 2).

Of the departments from the 73 respondent medical schools (48 responding department chairs and 25 responding practice plans), 57

---

[12] Paradoxically, while the department is at a significant financial disadvantage in treating Medicaid patients under the structure of the practice plan, teaching hospitals in many parts of the country are now competing heavily for these patients (because of more favorable reimbursement rates than managed care). In these settings, the department's financial problems are being compounded by the hospital's own efforts to increase Medicaid activity. A hospital CEO chastising the department in this circumstance for its lack of profitability seems unfair.

participate in organized faculty practice plans. Of the 57 schools with centralized plans, 64% indicated that their practice plan has established "discipline specific standards of productivity." It is not clear how these standards are being implemented, but in the case studies (where more information was necessarily available) departmental productivity is still being judged on the basis of the departmental financial bottom line and not on the basis of individual and group measures of specialty-based parameters of clinical productivity. In this context, the psychiatry department may not be able to offer incentives to individuals for exceptional cost-effective clinical performance from clinical revenue surpluses, because the department (unlike some specialties) does not have credible surpluses from its clinical activity (professional fee billing).

Table 1–6 outlines the patterns of charges that practice plans allocate to departments of psychiatry. Only a minority of practice plans appear to be billing departments for administrative services such as billing and collections and medical records on the basis of number of transactions. The actual percentage of total charges or percentage of net revenue used to calculate the allocated charges by practice plans to departments varied widely. Yet, as described in the Stanford case, the allocated charges can mean the difference between a department that is breaking even and a

TABLE 1-6

Practice plan charges allocated to departments of psychiatry as represented by 57 responding departments or practice plans

	Number of departments charged on the basis of			
Type of allocated charge	Percentage of total charges	Percentage of net revenue	Number of transactions	Actual cost
Bad debts and allowances	9	6	2	30
Billing and collections	12	27	3	11
Managed care and marketing	6	16	0	4
Malpractice	8	7	0	28
Space	8	9	0	21
Medical records	3	8	4	9
Physician extenders	2	2	0	25
Nonseparated charges	1	6	0	0
Other	5	8	0	8

department in deficit. Indeed, as the case examples from Stanford and Colorado illustrate, departments may be paying for central administrative services such as managed care marketing for the practice, but the practice may be failing to provide the department with relevant assistance in securing managed behavioral health contracts.

The general limitations for psychiatry in the most common information system employed by faculty practice plans (IDX) are highlighted in the University of Maryland case report. The fact that this information system has been used so widely across faculty practices for many years, without its software engineers being obliged to respond to these deficiencies, should be of concern to practice plan managers as well as psychiatry departments. Currently 17 of the 48 departments that responded to the question of capitation are participating in capitated contracts. For most of these (all but three), it represents a very small percentage of clinical income. It is unclear how risk would be assumed within the practice plan and hospital for the psychiatry department if capitation were to become a more significant factor for psychiatry departments.

When general tertiary-care hospitals budget in usual and customary ways, psychiatric beds may be considered a net loss because they are allocated the indirect costs of ancillary services but do not generate much activity for the operating room or radiology suite. When bed charges for psychiatry in the teaching hospital are similar to the charges on medicine and surgery, it is impossible for the psychiatry program to compete against comparable programs in community general hospitals and freestanding psychiatric hospitals. If the teaching hospital produces a competitive rate for psychiatric bed charges by reducing or eliminating the indirect costs of ancillary services, the teaching hospital will have to adjust its internal cost structures in ways that will affect other clinical departments.

Within the principal teaching hospital, 24 of 38 respondent departments receive some funding for "medical direction." Twelve of the respondent departments have recently downsized their inpatient capacity to accommodate the new managed care environment. Half of the respondent departments believe that the bed charges for psychiatry at the principal teaching hospital are "not competitive" enough to secure essential managed care business. More than twice as many of the respondent departments reported that their hospitals calculate the profitability of psychiatric beds to include the allocation of indirect costs for all hospital services rather than on the basis of direct costs only. By these criteria, psychiatry must consistently be unprofitable.

Of the 68 schools on which we have data on a dean's tax, 65 departments of psychiatry pay such a tax based on a percentage of gross revenue or net revenue from clinical or gross income. If based on a percentage of gross billings, departments may be disadvantaged where collections have been reduced by increases in the Medicaid population, increased indigent care, or substantial growth in discounted fee-for-service activity from managed care.

Although the data are necessarily incomplete, there appears to be little question that as most academic health centers experience substantial and multifaceted financial pressures, academic psychiatry departments could be very seriously affected because of the vulnerability of clinical and public-sector income and the uncertainties of grant-related income. While these issues are present in many academic clinical departments, the unique problems posed by behavioral health exclusions and the mixed financial blessing of psychiatry's recent success in securing federal research support contribute to the palpable feelings of anxiety among psychiatry faculty at a number of academic health centers.

Summary

This text highlights the ways academic departments of psychiatry are attempting to reconfigure their clinical (Chapter 2) and educational (Chapter 3) programs to accommodate the demands of managed care on the department and its parent academic health center. In addition to presenting data on what departments are doing, the reports also describe other options that they might consider to cope more effectively with the present crisis. Chapter 4 discusses some of the ways departments are funding the essential infrastructure for research on psychiatric and addictive disorders. As described here and also in Chapter 4, research has been one of the most exciting developments in psychiatry in the past two decades.

Chapter 5 describes the complex interface and opportunities for psychiatry and primary care. Although historically these disciplines have not generally been collaborative, the times call for cooperative innovations that will benefit patient care, education, and clinical and health services research in the areas of general and mental health. Chapter 6 describes changes in the programs under the Department of Veterans Affairs, which is increasingly recognizing that veterans carry the scars of their experiences in a high rate of mental and addictive disorders. The VA could be a model for linking academic and public-sector programs under a managed care model.

Chapter 7 presents an overview of the six cases and summarizes their lessons for psychiatry and academic health centers in general. It includes a summary of recommendations to the field that are bound to generate some controversy. The bottom-line message is that the times call for significant changes in the practice and teaching of psychiatry. If the field can be supported to implement significant change, the lessons learned will be helpful to psychiatry and to other areas of the academic clinical enterprise in the United States.

References

Billi JE, Wise CG, Bills EA, et al: Potential effects of managed care on specialty practice at a university medical center. N Engl J Med 333:979–983, 1995

Frank RG, McGuire TG: Estimating costs of mental health and substance abuse coverage. Health Affairs 14:102–115, 1995

Iglehart JK: Rapid changes for academic medical centers. N Engl J Med 331:1391–1395, 1994

Iglehart JK: Rapid changes for academic medical centers, II. N Engl J Med 332:407–411, 1995

Institute of Medicine, Division of Health Sciences Policy, Committee on Policies for Allocating Health Sciences Research Funds: Funding Health Sciences Research: A Strategy to Restore Balance, Washington, DC, National Academy Press, 1990

Jonas HS, Etzel SI, Barzansky B: Educational programs in US medical schools. JAMA 266:913–920, 1991

Kassirer JP: Academic medical centers under siege. N Engl J Med 331:1370–1371, 1994

Oss ME: Managed Behavioral Health Market Share in the United States, 1994. Gettysburg, PA, OPEN MINDS, June 1994

Talbott JA, Lomax JW, Beresin EV, et al: The impact of economic and health care delivery changes on psychiatric residency training. Proceedings of the American Association of Chairmen of Departments of Psychiatry Conference, Baltimore, MD, August 1995

University Hospital Consortium: Competing in the Maturing Health Care Marketplace: Strategies for Academic Medical Centers, Vol 1. Chicago, IL, University Hospital Consortium, 1993

Wiener JP: Forecasting the effects of health reform on US physician workforce requirements: evidence from HMO staffing patterns. JAMA 272:222–230, 1994

CHAPTER 2

The Response of Academic Psychiatry to Managed Care: Clinical Delivery Systems

Roger E. Meyer, M.D., and Christopher J. McLaughlin

Academic psychiatry departments face extremely complicated choices as they confront changes in the health care delivery system. Although some general tactics are important for academic psychiatry departments to consider as they attempt to shape their clinical services to meet the requirements of managed care, there is no single strategy that will work for all (or most) departments. Each department will need to craft a strategy shaped by its clinical capacity and expertise, the opportunities in the public sector, local private-sector demand, the strategic direction of the parent academic health center, the entrepreneurial spirit and attitudes among department faculty and the leadership of the overall clinical delivery system, the stage of evolution of the faculty practice arrangements, the maturity of the health insurance market relative to managed care penetration, and the attitudes in other clinical departments and the academic health center (AHC) administration toward psychiatry (and psychiatrists).

Managed behavioral health care companies also differ in a number of ways from each other.[1] While some of the initial leadership in the industry was clinically sophisticated, a succession of mergers and acquisitions has shifted the ownership of some of the leading companies to for-profit hospital chains, large health maintenance organizations (HMOs), or Wall Street deal makers. As price competition between the companies has intensified, the discounted fee-for-service and capitation rates offered to providers have raised questions about the availability of appropriate levels of care for the chronic and seriously mentally ill, as well as the disproportionate rationing of health care to this population (compared with the general health sector) (Jellinek and Nurcombe 1993). The carveouts have also raised important questions regarding the potential fragmentation of care: 1) How can integrated health care services be delivered to persons with chronic illness in the context of carveouts of portions of health care delivery? 2) How have the total health care needs of patients with mental or addictive disorders been integrated in the context of the behavioral health carveout? Answers to these questions are yet to be determined. Advocates of the carveout strategy argue that instead of psychotherapeutic care being focused on a relatively small number of "worried well," managed behavioral health care can assure that appropriate levels of care will be available to more people in need (Boyle and Callahan 1995).

In this chapter we examine the options open to academic departments of psychiatry (and their parent institutions) in this age of managed behavioral health care. We believe that the proper course for academic psychiatry in these times is to advocate for and deliver the highest quality clinical services to the seriously mentally ill and to assure integrated psychosocial and behavioral health services for patients in the general and specialized health care programs of the AHC. The leaders of academic medicine and psychiatry also need to recognize that even if academic psychiatry departments can evolve into, or become part of, behavioral health systems, there is no certainty that they will be able to subsidize their academic mission from clinical income. The case example from Sheppard and Enoch Pratt Health System describes the successful evo-

---

[1] The recent relatively high rate of turnover in ownership and management has complicated the ability of providers (including AHCs) to develop working relationships or joint ventures with the companies.

lution of a psychiatric hospital into a behavioral health system that cannot afford its traditional graduate medical education (GME) program.[2]

The managed care unit, described in the case report from the University of Colorado, has been removed from residency and undergraduate medical education programs and does not generate a financial surplus from operations. Ultimately, even departments that can change their clinical programs to meet the requirements of the marketplace will need to assess their educational and research missions and develop cost-effective strategies for these efforts (including local and regional collaboration). Clinical income will not cover the underfunded costs of education and research in psychiatry. Moreover, because of a number of problems that complicate cost-efficient psychiatric practice in some faculty practice plans, some departments may choose to minimize their clinical involvement in intensively managed care settings to focus on research and teaching (Stanford case report).

The goal of a focused effort to increase managed behavioral health business should be to enable the department's clinical programs to remain financially sound in the context of discounted fee-for-service or capitated contracts. The traditional psychodynamically oriented models of long-term psychotherapeutic care that flourished in some centers are irrelevant to the world of managed behavioral health care (even though medical educators and primary care physicians and training programs continue to value teaching, which increases understanding of patients' behavior and communication, and even though some patients are willing to pay for these services out of pocket). For psychotherapists to remain skilled as educators, they must be able to practice their art, even if it means that the academic practice loses money.[3]

Although no department can support a predominantly psychotherapy-based faculty practice in these times, neither should it be forced to abandon a psychotherapy service of limited size. As I describe near the end of this chapter, for academic psychiatry to develop its full potential

---

[2] The latter is being merged with the psychiatric residency training program at the University of Maryland.

[3] Teachers of brief dynamic psychotherapy need to be able to continue to do some long-term psychotherapy to maintain their skills with brief and long-term modalities of treatment.

in its clinical practice, it will require a support structure that can successfully exploit the entrepreneurial opportunities extant in the field (the opportunities beyond fee-for-service psychotherapy).

The Context

In general, one can discern three stages in the evolution of behavioral health care carveouts across the country. The three stages are not necessarily inevitable or sequential, since not all programs have evolved to the same degree. Indeed, all three stages may be present at the same time in the same community. In the first stage, a self-insured employer, HMO, or insurance company contracts with a managed behavioral health care company to offer services to all members with mental or addictive disorders. The latter company contracts with a selected group of local providers on a discounted fee-for-service basis. Because of a surplus of mental health service providers in many communities, the company places pressure on individual professionals and hospitals for steep discounts. In fact, with each succeeding year, those pressures may result in larger discounts. Providers who make use of psychiatric hospital beds to a "disproportionate" degree (relative to treatment in less-expensive venues) are dropped from the provider pool.

In the second stage of evolution, the behavioral health carveout company invites local providers to assume "risk" in capitated contracts, which are analogous to the contracts that the carveout company has with an HMO or insurance company. The carveout company has gained experience with the practice patterns of its local provider network and initiates the move to shift the financial risk from itself to the provider group. Some behavioral health care executives have raised ethical questions about this type of arrangement (Gold et al. 1995). In some parts of Southern California, providers are paid $0.50–$0.75 per member per month (PMPM) for behavioral health services for clients (not including the costs of hospitalization) (S. Feldman, personal communication, December 1995). The difference between the capitation rate paid to the carveout company and the capitation rate paid to the provider group covers the costs of program administration.

Extremely low capitation rates for behavioral health services are not compatible with the treatment needs of chronically and severely mentally ill and addicted patients and constitute a perverse incentive to families of mentally ill patients to sign up with other plans that offer more realistic mental health benefits. This practice is called *adverse selection* and can lead to the concentration of more costly mental health care in more responsible managed behavioral health care plans (Frank et al. 1996). Moreover, because of the acknowledged expertise of some psychiatry faculty in the treatment of complex mental disorders, the adverse selection strategies of less-responsible managed behavioral health care companies exclude the faculty members from some provider networks.

The third stage of evolution of managed behavioral health care is much less developed in most communities. In some settings, provider groups have determined that if they contract directly with payers or corporations for behavioral health services, they can eliminate the costs of the insurance company or HMO and the behavioral health carveout company. This type of initiative means that the provider organization has some of the characteristics of an insurance entity (or the initiative can be a joint venture with an insurance company). Sheppard-Pratt has, in fact, been able to develop these functions while retaining its other discounted fee-for-service and capitated contracts with managed behavioral health care companies. Few if any academic psychiatry departments are positioned to undertake this type of effort. However, in the context of possible congressional action authorizing physician-owned entities and hospitals to compete with insurance companies and HMOs for direct corporate contracts, this newly recognized role could become an opportunity for new or joint ventures for teaching (and teaching-affiliated) hospitals, faculty practice plans, and affiliated faculty.

The Challenge

If the clinical service and graduate medical education programs offered by academic psychiatry departments are to compete in a discounted fee-for-service or capitated managed care environment, they will need to 1) bring down hospital bed charges to community standards; 2) reduce average lengths of stay on inpatient units to less than 7 days; 3) focus inpatient care to stabilize patients and prepare them for transfer to less-intensive venues of treatment; 4) be able to access (or implement their own) partial hospital/intensive outpatient and nonhospital residential programs; 5) offer goal-oriented treatment at all levels; 6) implement a strong quality assurance or utilization review program that monitors clinician performance in relation to functional patient outcomes; 7) emphasize brief psychotherapies, excellence in pharmacotherapy management, and the ability to diagnose and treat comorbid mental and addictive disorders; 8) develop a geographically distributed, cost-effective, high-quality, and multidisciplinary ambulatory care delivery system; and 9) attempt to integrate educational programs into managed care contracts.

The marketing of behavioral health services and the development of a geographically distributed network of community-based mental health service providers require special expertise that may not be present within departments of psychiatry or faculty practice plans, but they are critical to success. The overall effort would be strengthened by the availability of actuarial expertise in the negotiations with managed care organizations and by a solid information system for internal cost analysis and reporting purposes.

Table 2–1 lists the initiatives being made by the respondent departments to accommodate their practice patterns to the requirements of managed behavioral health care. Because each of the respondents was asked to list up to five initiatives, the frequency of responses reflected in the table may be related to the perceived importance of specific tactics and strategies or the relative ease of implementation across departments. From 44 departments, 187 responses were received (4.25 responses per department). More than 50% of the departments have modified or developed alternatives to inpatient care, implemented an internal utilization review program, or reshaped the ambulatory care service to accommodate the requirements of managed care organizations. Of the 44 departments, 11 are providing contractual utilization review for managed care companies. The clinical care systems of between 20% and 25% of the respondents have been redirected (in part) to incorporate a case management system, nonphysician clinicians, or a community provider network. Five of the respondents have replaced nontenured clinicians with contract employees. Improved marketing and faculty de-

TABLE 2-1

Practice responses to managed care reported by 44 departments

Managed care response	Number of departments responding
Modify or develop alternatives to inpatient service	25
Internal utilization review	24
Reshape ambulatory care service	23
Prepare new clinical program initiatives	16
Develop community provider network	13
Hire nonphysician clinicians	12
Contractual utilization review for managed care companies	11
Improve marketing	9
Faculty development	9
Develop case management system	9
Work with university-managed care program	7
Reconfigure or develop alternatives to emergency room service	5
Eliminate nontenured clinicians or shift to contract employees	5
Establish health maintenance or managed care organization	4
Provide Medicaid care	3
Provide psychiatric services in primary care sites	3
Develop new administrative structures	3
Restructure resident service delivery	3
No department response to managed care	2
Acquire clinical service entity	1

velopment were each cited by approximately 20% of the respondents as important to their efforts to accommodate managed care.

As described in the case reports from Maryland and Colorado, some departments have created distinct managed care–oriented clinical programs or divisions. In some ways, this type of effort is analogous to the creation of the Saturn Corporation by General Motors, where the parent company decided that creating a new operating entity was more cost-effective than attempting to change the corporate culture as a whole. In contrast, the case report from Dartmouth describes an effort to transform the total clinical (and residency training programs) of the department so that it might better serve the needs of its parent health care delivery system—as well as its own position—in relationship to managed care. Although the strategies chosen by the leadership at Dartmouth were different than those developed at Maryland and Colorado, each of the efforts acknowledged the urgency of change, and the cultural resistance to change, within an academic department.

Since only 17 departments reported participation in capitated contracts, and only 3 of these showed significant clinical income from this activity, it would appear that most of the income from managed care activities is from discounted fee-for-service programs. In many places, the authority to accept financial risk in capitated behavioral health contracts may be too far removed (in the hospital and faculty practice plan) from the psychiatry department that has responsibility for delivering services within a fixed budget. The distribution of profits or losses from such ventures may not yet be clearly worked out in faculty practice plans that have not fully evolved into multispecialty groups. Most psychiatry departments' budgets are too marginal to handle the financial risk of capitation.

A more satisfactory approach to capitation or the negotiation of case rates for care would bring together hospital and professional charges and risk sharing. The case examples from Sheppard-Pratt and the University of Colorado highlight the importance of managing psychiatric services through a single revenue center that brings together professional fees and charges for all venues of care. Since faculty practice plans, by definition, are only empowered to address the professional fee side of the equation, academic health centers (practice plans and teaching hospitals) might work together with the leadership of their academic psychiatry departments to create an administrative structure that can offer a single point of negotiation for managed behavioral health care.[4]

The contrast between departments of psychiatry that can and cannot make decisions about managed behavioral health care is highlighted in the following quotation from the chair at the University of California–San Francisco (UCSF)/Langley Porter Hospital and Clinics (C. Van Dyke, personal communication, March 1996): "The great advantage that I enjoy is that I am able to make decisions about Langley Porter and our mental health business. . . . The Medical Center had major issues of its

---

[4] As described near the end of this chapter, the optimal structure is most likely to evolve in those academic health centers where there is clinical product line development and management and where behavioral health services can be developed as a distinct product line.

own and was unable to devote the necessary time and energy to helping us. . . . I have assumed the authority and . . . I am the person on campus who . . . is in a position to make decisions about mental health. . . . I have been able to move much more rapidly than the overall clinical enterprise."

Langley Porter has its own marketing and contracting individual within the marketing and contracting office of the medical center. Half of the salary comes from Langley Porter. The administrative structure has facilitated the negotiation of behavioral health carveouts as the preferred provider for at least one major company, a goal that has been more difficult to implement at nearby Stanford, where the department is embedded in a more or less traditional faculty practice plan. The medical director at U.S. Behavioral Health (USBH)[5] Company, Dr. William Goldman, agrees that the delegated authority and support structures available to the psychiatry department at UCSF account in large measure for its contractual success (personal communication, March 1996). Indeed, the structure at UCSF has enabled the department of psychiatry to develop a number of joint programs with U.S. Behavioral Health.

One of the real success stories in changing a clinical service delivery system has occurred at Northwestern University. Since 1991, when Dr. Sheldon Miller became chair, the psychiatry department has continued to derive approximately 80% of its funding from clinical service revenue, but that annual income has gone from $5.4 million to $13.5 million. According to Dr. Miller (personal communication, October 1996), the department operates in an environment with many aspects of a true multispecialty practice ethic. Interdepartmental clinical centers of excellence work well and have incorporated active liaison services from the psychiatry department. These interconnections serve to provide quality assurance of psychosocial services throughout the health care delivery system at Northwestern. The psychiatry department also benefits from referrals for consultation and treatment from throughout the hospital and practice plan. There is a developing consultation-liaison (CL) service to ambulatory primary care sites. The department has evolved from one made up principally of part-time clinicians supported

---

[5] Now called United Behavioral Health.

by medical administrative dollars from the hospital to a group of full-time faculty and a broad network of affiliated clinicians across the greater Chicago area. The job descriptions of clinically active faculty now focus on full-time responsibility for revenue generation and the academic mission rather than a singular focus on a part-time hospital position. Funding to the department from the hospital continues to be an important source of faculty support.

When Dr. Miller arrived, the hospital already owned a managed behavioral health care company with less than 100,000 covered lives through subcontracts with major insurers in the Chicago area. Between 1991 and 1996, the number of covered lives grew to 450,000. Dr. Miller believes that the company has been profitable for the hospital, offsetting losses related to psychiatric beds and the costs of medical administration across the span of hospital-based psychiatric services. The department has been able to develop capitated contracts with the managed behavioral health company, ranging from full psychiatric services to simple administrative oversight of behavioral health benefits. The department's relationship with the managed behavioral health company has enabled it to develop its network of community-based providers and to provide patients for its own faculty. Apart from the hospital's managed behavioral health care company, the practice plan and hospital also collaborate in managed care contracting, which has been relevant to psychiatry.

Finally, while the faculty practice plan structure at Northwestern does not pool its revenues and expenses across departments as in a multispecialty group practice, the plan holds the department responsible for a "realistic" level of planned deficit in income versus expenses. The goals for psychiatry are based on discipline-specific standards of productivity—as in a multispecialty practice group. With regard to these standards, the department has developed an information system that tracks productivity and performs internal utilization review in support of its managed care contracts. The department also includes forensic work as part of its practice plan activities. This type of clinical income is taxed at a lower rate than other clinical income—and helps make up for the heavily discounted fees from managed care and Medicaid.

If an academic psychiatry department is to participate in behavioral health carveouts, its parent practice plan and teaching hospital will need to work with the psychiatry department chair to address problems of cost, cost-allocation methods, and support structure. The chair may need the support of the medical center to develop a network of community-based masters-prepared clinicians, doctoral-level psychologists, and psychiatrists for whom the AHC would become the contracting agent in discounted fee-for-service and capitated contracts. If these individuals were employed by the department, they would substantially increase its expenses through the fixed costs of salaries and fringe benefits. The department could become the provider of continuing clinical education for these service providers to strengthen their practice skills in a managed care environment. The leadership in psychiatry should seek to bind individual clinicians to the network through a common information system and performance-based contracts and be responsible for quality assurance and utilization review within the practice network. At this juncture, it is not clear whether the network strategies identified by 13 of the respondent departments (Table 2–1) have been amplified by these types of efforts.

In some places, psychiatry faculty will need to be retooled to practice in a cost-sensitive manner. As shown in Table 2–1, 20% of the responding departments have embarked on a program of faculty development to prepare practicing clinicians to work more effectively with patients under the rules set down by managed behavioral health care organizations. In a recent personal communication (August 1996) and in frequent public statements, Dr. William Goldman of U.S. Behavioral Health has listed the qualities of psychiatrists preferred by his organization. USBH prefers practitioners who are competent in the delivery of validated brief psychotherapies and values psychiatrists who are comfortable treating patients with dual mental illness and substance abuse problems. The company presumes that psychiatrists should be uniquely qualified to deliver psychotherapy and pharmacotherapy in an integrated manner[6] and to offer medication backup to other mental health professionals delivering psychotherapy.

---

[6] Regrettably, the reality is that, under the extremely low capitation or discounted fee-for-service rates offered by some of the managed behavioral health companies, it has become financially untenable for psychiatrists to provide psychotherapy. Dr. Goldman of USBH believes that integrated psychotherapy and pharmacotherapy by a psychiatrist is more cost-effective than care delivered by two or more professionals.

Psychiatry faculty need to manifest attitudes of service and accountability. They will need to maintain responsibility for treatment outcome based on measurable functional improvement and lengthened periods of remission in patients who continue to carry their initial diagnoses or risks of relapse. The integration of general and behavioral health services for patients with chronic mental or addictive disorders would be advanced by psychiatrists who can serve the basic medical care needs of this population directly or in collaborative arrangements with primary care clinicians.

The managed care contracts office for the practice plan and hospital will need to assure that the psychiatry department that has been organized to participate in managed behavioral health care is included in comprehensive contracts for managed health care. As described in the case reports from Colorado and Louisville, because so much of managed behavioral health care has been carved out to for-profit companies that exclude academic psychiatry departments, some academic medical centers have been obliged to *exclude* colleagues in psychiatry from contracts for general health care services provided by faculty. Based on a separate informal survey, the practice may be fairly widespread. In addition to the patent unfairness and economic disadvantages to the psychiatry department in these arrangements, the contracts make it very difficult to deliver integrated health services to patients who require psychiatric consultation or intervention. In some places, even contracts covering health care to university employees have proscribed access to the university's own faculty psychiatrists (B. Eichelman, personal communication, January 1996).

If, as a consequence of these carveouts, the psychiatry department is unable to gain access to the managed care activity that has been contracted to the rest of the medical center, the hospital, school, and practice plan may need to assist the department financially and in other ways to make up for the loss of clinical revenue. As described in a later section, the department of psychiatry has a number of options in assisting the medical center to deal more effectively with managed care for general and specialized health services. The department could be compensated by the medical center for these efforts and might be subsidized at somewhat higher levels for its teaching activities.

Psychiatric Practice in the Service of the Academic Health Center: Primary Care

Where an academic health center has been organized to serve *all* of the health care needs of a population under capitated arrangements (or under its own HMO), specialty services (including psychiatry) are usually accessed through a primary care gatekeeper who may have incentive to provide most of this care herself or himself.[7] If behavioral health services can be accessed only through a gatekeeper, psychiatry faculty may be best positioned as part of the primary care health care delivery team (see Chapter 5). Here they can serve more effectively as consultants and providers of acute care, and the department of psychiatry is thus positioned to assist the academic health center in demonstrable ways. Craig Van Dyke, the chair at UCSF/Langley Porter, has also highlighted this issue: "Because of (our) separate history, (we) never provided the types of clinical services that the rest of the Medical Center expected of us. . . . We have (now) made a major effort to become more relevant, particularly in outpatient consultation and in being a full-fledged partner in the carved-in Health Net business that applies to the whole medical center" (personal communication, March 1996).

The major issues in the boundary between psychiatry and primary care are discussed at length in Chapter 5. The resources necessary to develop closely linked clinical programs are beyond the usual financial capabilities of primary care and psychiatry departments, unless they are subsidized by the AHC and/or teaching hospital. As the institution attempts to transform itself into an integrated health care delivery system in a competitive environment, the development of a cost-efficient primary care system will be enhanced if patients with mental disorders or subthreshold psychiatric conditions can receive prompt assessment and appropriate consultation and treatment in the primary care setting.

---

[7] We are aware of at least one exception to this model. The George Washington University Health Plan contracted with its academic psychiatry department to "carve out" behavioral health services for a portion of the enrollees in the HMO. The latter could access the mental health provider directly, without referral from a primary care clinician. However, the capitation rate was double community standards and for other members of the HMO, where the primary care physicians served as gatekeepers. The HMO did not like the model, and it is unlikely to continue in the future.

Specialty Psychiatric Care in the Academic Health Center

Within the tertiary/quaternary care programs and centers of clinical excellence of many academic health centers, there may be another important role for academic psychiatry. In most places, there has been little effort made to coordinate an approach to the organization and delivery of psychosocial services. Hospital social service departments may report to senior financial or administrative officers rather than to the offices that oversee patient services. Separate programs of clinical excellence (e.g., cancer center, cardiac center, women's health center, physical medicine, and rehabilitation) may bypass the psychiatry department and the hospital social service department in hiring their own staff of psychologists and social workers. In general, these arrangements appear to shield psychosocial service programs from an overall examination of quality assurance and potential cost savings related to patient care. As described in the case study from Dartmouth, multidisciplinary diagnostic and treatment teams within the psychiatry department can reach out to other specialized care systems within an AHC to offer a single point of accountability for the quality and cost of psychosocial and behavioral health services.

Although the consultation-liaison services of some academic psychiatry departments might be well-positioned to provide this type of service within their academic health centers, many CL services are focused almost exclusively on bedside consultations. In this regard, they present problems of access and limited clinical capacity to the rest of the medical center and ambulatory practice areas. The contrast between Dartmouth and Northwestern on the one hand, and some of the other case report departments on the other hand, suggests that multispecialty group practice modes of governance and operations within a faculty practice plan may be more supportive of coordinated psychosocial services than are traditional departmental or federated practice plan structures.

In an optimal environment, the academic psychiatry department could be charged by AHC and clinical program leadership with cost-reduction and quality-enhancement targets for psychosocial services.

With many centers of clinical excellence now using inpatient and multiple ambulatory settings for care (e.g., comprehensive cancer centers), this type of effort represents a logistical challenge, but the Dartmouth case study highlights the feasibility of utilizing a broad cadre of mental health professionals in this effort. A number of studies have demonstrated that psychiatric consultation can help to reduce lengths of stay on surgical inpatient units and overall health care utilization (Holder and Hallan 1986; Schlesinger et al. 1983). Because fees for these services, performed by a psychiatrist or other mental health professional, may not be adequately reimbursed in intensively managed care settings, their costs may need to be bundled with other charges. Under this arrangement, the psychiatry department would be reimbursed by its hospital or practice plan from fees collected.

Managed Care, the Public Sector, and Academic Psychiatry

As described in Chapter 4, as well as in the case reports from the University of Louisville, the University of Colorado, the University of Maryland, and Dartmouth, a number of academic psychiatry departments continue to benefit substantially from their collaboration with public-sector mental health and addiction programs. At a time when the private sector offers diminishing opportunities for residency graduates because of the impact of managed care, the public sector continues to serve as a virtual reservoir of employment opportunities for interested psychiatrists.

On the other side of the coin, a number of states have begun privatizing Medicaid. In some areas, this shift has resulted in perverse incentives for some managed care companies. In Philadelphia, the Commonwealth of Pennsylvania was paying $30 PMPM to HMOs for behavioral health services (B. Eichelman, personal communication, January 1996). The HMOs contracted with behavioral health companies for $15 PMPM to provide these services. The difference between $15 and $30 covered the HMOs' "administrative costs," making this program highly profitable for them. The managed behavioral health companies contracted with local providers at discounted fee-for-service rates for the treatment of individuals with mental or addictive disorders. Since at any given time only 5%–6% of the Medicaid population was in mental health or addiction treatment, the behavioral health companies also found this program quite profitable. None of the academic psychiatry departments in Philadelphia were apparently positioned to contract directly with the HMOs for the capitated behavioral health carveout. Clinical programs in some of the academic psychiatry departments in the city participated in discounted fee-for-service arrangements with behavioral health carve-out companies but found them financially less favorable than the old Medicaid program that heavily discounted fees to psychiatrists. In some of the programs, the volume of Medicaid patients declined. At this writing, it is unclear whether the city will be empowered to correct problems in the program and move to a fully capitated carveout of behavioral health services.

It seems clear that as states gain experience with these programs, they will be obliged to price them to reduce the profitability experienced by HMOs and behavioral health companies in Philadelphia. A number of communities may see accelerated closings of state hospitals. In Maryland, community mental health centers (CMHCs) will be competing with for-profit behavioral health companies for Medicaid and public-sector patients. At least some of these CMHCs are university related. It would appear that in a number of states, Medicaid and the public mental health care system are being brought together in managed behavioral health programs, partially because the for-profit managed behavioral health care companies have targeted this area as a major growth opportunity.

Academic psychiatry department faculty and their colleagues in the public sector need to combine resources to develop high-quality and cost-effective carveout strategies for these populations. Failure to anticipate the potential loss of the remaining linkages between public-sector and academic psychiatry would represent a major loss to academic psychiatry. If states shift to managed behavioral health care companies to direct the care of former public-sector and Medicaid patients with chronic mental and addictive disorders, academic psychiatry departments will have to work with the companies to maintain their involvement with this patient population. If the report from Philadelphia is a harbinger of what is to come, academic departments should be concerned.

Mental Disorders as Paradigms for Chronic Disease Management

As academic health centers attempt to cope with the new world of managed care, there is a growing appreciation among the press and the public in some locations that a cost-efficient health care delivery system may actually mean withholding care for some individuals (Brook et al. 1996; Hoffman et al. 1996). It was recently reported that while population-based health care tends to serve the needs of healthy and acutely ill individuals reasonably well, individuals with chronic illnesses may face limitations on coverage for services that might compromise their care (Newhouse 1994). This study appeared to confirm the impressions of some policy analysts: "Although from 80 to 85% of illnesses and disability involves chronic conditions, . . . the acute care oriented US health system has not come to grips with these needs. . . . Due to adverse risk selection, the health care system has incentives for avoiding provision of services to persons with chronic conditions. . . . While (there are) opportunities for management and coordination of services . . . for chronic conditions . . . the opportunities are not being pursued" (The George Washington University National Health Policy Forum, unpublished observations, November 1995).

The issue is also of concern for children with chronic illnesses: "Health care for children with chronic illnesses is significantly more expensive than for the average child. Children with chronic illnesses are especially vulnerable in a competitive health care environment because of the higher costs associated with treating their illnesses and the inherent pressures to reduce services to manage within the capitated rate"[8] (Neff and Anderson 1995, p. 1868). The reports dealing with chronic illness in the managed care environment have suggested changes in models of managed care reimbursement to account for the higher costs associated with the treatment and management of chronic illnesses. Suggestions include capitated carveouts for specific medical conditions, with capitated pricing rates that would reflect the higher costs associated with the illness (Fowles et al. 1996), or the implementation of a retrospective

---

[8] While this report focused on children with nonpsychiatric chronic illnesses, the same issues pertain to children with chronic psychiatric conditions.

risk adjuster (The George Washington University National Health Policy Forum, unpublished observations, November 1995). As the latter paper noted, "Health plans and systems are searching for solutions, and none is readily apparent."

In fairness, there were also problems for the chronically ill under traditional fee-for-service medicine, where patterns of reimbursement favored those who provided high-tech acute diagnostic and interventional care. The complex costs of care stemming from chronic illness and disability were often left to the welfare system or some other safety net provider. Patients with severe disabilities consequent to chronic illness might end up outside of the private health insurance system in Medicare and Medicaid. Many of the real costs of disability could be linked only indirectly to health care. The ancillary costs of care, such as patient education and case management to enhance treatment compliance, were not covered under fee-for-service models of specialist reimbursement. It is not clear how these needs are being met in the cost-focused primary care–managed care environment.

The psychiatrist David Reiss has described the dilemma: "Modern medicine has changed dying patients into chronic patients" (D. Reiss, personal communication, April 1994). Traditionally, persons with disabilities consequent to chronic illnesses have been served by specialized providers of care. The specialty mission of academic medicine does not involve only complex organ transplants but also the advancement of knowledge and care, by specialists, to individuals with chronic diseases. Although it is clear that we do not need as many specialists as we have been producing, we will continue to need the knowledge generated by specialists who can foster innovation in patient care through research.

Academic health centers should be well positioned to articulate and serve the needs of patients with chronic illnesses through disease-management strategies. Academic departments of psychiatry have a special responsibility to articulate and serve the needs of chronic and severely mentally ill and addicted patients. As academic health centers begin to invest in disease-management strategies,[9] they may rethink their

---

[9] Curiously, some pharmaceutical companies have invested resources in the development of disease-management products—but this effort seems more suited to AHCs.

traditional focus on tertiary and quaternary acute care. If managed care health plans find more incentive in minimizing their financial risks through case and provider selection, academic health centers can attempt to regain the moral high ground by developing cost-efficient systems of care for persons with chronic illnesses. Capitation rates need to be realistic and foster innovation. Community-based capitation rates for health care in which the vast majority of the population is healthy are not sufficient to address the needs of persons with chronic illnesses. The absurdly low capitated carveout rates for behavioral health services in Southern California ($0.50–$0.75 PMPM) are an extreme example of the problem.

Patient care needs to be cost and outcome sensitive. Outcomes must be judged on the basis of improved function, quality of life, and duration of remission from active symptoms and illness. In an optimal world, the capitation rate should foster a clinical environment in which new knowledge can be generated to improve treatment in the future. Because an appropriate methodology for calculating capitation rates for specific chronic illnesses does not now exist (The George Washington University Health Policy Forum 1995), academic health centers might develop and advocate for realistic needs-based capitation for some of the more common chronic illnesses. In the context of public sector–academic collaborations, appropriately capitated carveouts focusing on the chronically mentally ill should provide such a model. As mentioned in the case report from Colorado, the public mental health authority in that state is working with the leadership of the academic department to develop one such needs-based formula for capitation of carved out services to the chronically mentally ill.

One Potential Structure for the Future Management of Clinical Programs in Academic Psychiatry

As described in the introductory section of this chapter, there can be no single clinical strategy that will meet the needs of all (or most) academic departments of psychiatry. As a general rule, the entrepreneurial possibilities for academic psychiatry are limited by the structure of clinical practice (hospitals and practice plans) within the parent academic health center. Centers that have evolved to clinical product line management from a departmental model appear to be in the best position to develop the entrepreneurial potential of academic psychiatry through focused direction of behavioral health services.[10] The goal of this effort can never be simply filling beds in the hospital. Such programs must strive for strong financial performance, and program elements should be consistent with the strengths and academic missions of specific departments of psychiatry.

Optimally, administrative support for behavioral health services would come from the hospital, the practice plan, and the department of psychiatry. The management team would be responsible for creating a budget-driven strategic plan for clinical services, as well as seeking out contracts with managed behavioral health care companies and developing potential joint ventures. The product line clinical program management would have to develop a geographically distributed network of community-based clinicians and oversee quality assurance of these clinicians and of full-time faculty in the department. A cornerstone of this effort might be the implementation of disease management strategies for mental and addictive disorders that are accountable for realistic functional outcomes.

Capitated or fee-for-service compensation would be based on reasonable expectations of service requirements of the patient population, as in the model being developed in Colorado. The implementation of a clinical trials program within this type of framework could dovetail with the interests of the pharmaceutical industry and with the need to continuously improve the treatment system. Finally, the behavioral health services system would be charged with oversight for all behavioral and

---

[10] None of the case study departments were operating in a pure product line–management environment. Vanderbilt University Medical Center is presently embarking on this strategy and includes a behavioral health product line among the 11 identified programs.

psychosocial services throughout the academic health center and its satellite and primary care locations. Appropriate cost and pricing of these services to the rest of the academic health center would necessarily be part of the initiative.

Apart from the academic health center, product line management would be responsible for negotiating contracts with the public sector to assure the best and most appropriate care for the chronic and severely mentally ill patients within the structure of a vital public sector–academic relationship. The disease-management strategies developed by clinical leadership within the behavioral health service program should work well with the developing interest of state governments in capitated models of care. Best practice would align these efforts with the work of advocacy and consumer groups for the mentally ill and their families. Another public-sector initiative that has been developed in some areas involves links between academic psychiatry and the criminal justice system. This union represents an opportunity for forensic psychiatrists, as well as for addiction psychiatrists working within the criminal justice system on treatment alternatives to sentencing.

Finally, as described in the case examples from Sheppard and Enoch Pratt and from the University of Maryland, there may be potential opportunities for some academic departments in working with (or offering) employee assistance programs to corporations in their areas. Occupational health programs offer a broad range of opportunities for well-positioned AHCs to work with their local corporate communities to advance treatment and prevention efforts under workers' compensation, health promotion, disease prevention, stress management, and drug and alcohol screening and treatment. This focus could help academic health centers attract corporate interest in their broader clinical programs, while generating goodwill among leading members of the business community. (The identity of some AHCs as their states' medical schools can foster the development of a broad array of employee assistance and health services programs for state employees.) These various occupational health programs could provide a valuable referral linkage between psychiatry and the rest of the clinical delivery system of the AHC in a way that might be analogous to the emerging role of primary care disciplines under managed care.

Summary

The historical organization of many academic health centers around the practice requirements of surgical, medical, and hospital-based specialists and subspecialists has generally worked to the disadvantage of clinical programs in psychiatry and primary care. In the current environment of managed care and intense competition, all academic health centers must struggle to find the funds to support the costs of education and research, to control the costs of clinical care, and to meet the health care needs of their communities (Korn 1996). As centers have begun to change in order to compete more effectively in the new health care environment, some of their leaders have come to appreciate the importance of primary care in the future clinical delivery system.

Now is also the time to rethink the place of psychiatry in this system. As a start, the leaders of AHCs and of academic psychiatry departments will need to think through the complexity of mission and the relevance of current administrative and cost structures affecting psychiatry. At a minimum, if an academic psychiatry department is to participate in behavioral health carveouts, its parent practice plan and teaching hospital will need to work with the department chair to address problems of cost, cost-allocation methods, and support structure. The department may also need assistance from the medical center to develop a network of community-based clinicians for whom the center would become the contracting agent in discounted fee-for-service and capitated contracts.

The direction of a behavioral health and psychosocial service system within an academic health center requires the same degree of specialized management expertise and operational authority as any other center of clinical excellence. Programmatically, meeting these needs will require an interdisciplinary model of patient care, including clinical psychologists, social workers, psychiatric nurses, occupational therapists, psychiatrists, and other physicians. Psychiatry departments succeeding in the new health care environment appear to operate without the types of structural problems of more typical practice plans, teaching hospitals, and universities. The elements of a successful model may be gleaned from the case studies from Dartmouth, Colorado, and Maryland and from a careful examination of the opportunities in clinical product line management of behavioral health services.

References

Boyle PJ, Callahan D: Managed care in mental health: the ethical issues. Health Affairs 14(suppl 3):7–22, 1995

Brook RH, Kamberg CJ, McGlynn EA: Health system reform and quality. JAMA 276:476–480, 1996

Fowles JB, Weiner JP, Knutson D, et al: Taking health status into account when setting capitation rates. JAMA 276:1316–1321, 1996

Frank RG, Haiden AH, McGuire TG, et al: Some economics of mental health carve-outs. Arch Gen Psychiatry 53:933–937, 1996

Hoffman C, Rice D, Sung H: Persons with chronic conditions: their prevalence and costs. JAMA 276:1473–1479, 1996

Holder HD, Hallan JB: Impact of alcoholism treatment on total health care costs: a six-year study. Advances in Alcoholism and Substance Abuse 6:1–15, 1986

Jellinek MS, Nurcombe B: Two wrongs don't make a right: managed care, mental health, and the marketplace. JAMA 274:1737–1739, 1993

Korn D: Reengineering academic health centers: reengineering academic values? Acad Med 71:1033–1043, 1996

Neff JM, Anderson G: Caring for the uninsured and underinsured: protecting children with chronic illness in a competitive marketplace. JAMA 274:1866–1869, 1995

Newhouse JP: Patients at risk: health reform and risk adjustment. Health Aff (Millwood) 13:132–146, 1994

Schlesinger HJ, Mumford E, Glass V, et al: Mental health treatment and medical care utilization in a fee-for-service system: outpatient mental health treatment following the onset of a chronic disease. Am J Public Health 73:422–429, 1983

CHAPTER 3

The Educational Missions of Academic Psychiatry

Roger E. Meyer, M.D., and Christopher J. McLaughlin

Among a series of major recommendations on the future of medical education in the United States, the Pew Commission on the Health Professions advocated that the undergraduate medical curriculum emphasize a biopsychosocial model of human health and illness (Pew Health Professions Commission 1995). The term *biopsychosocial* was coined by George Engel and highlighted in a seminal article in *Science* 20 years ago (Engel 1977). Engel's article was a response to the ideological schism in psychiatry between those who emphasized a medical model focusing on psychiatric disorders as brain disorders and those who argued that the field differed from the rest of medicine and should focus on individual psychology, psychodynamics, and the sociocultural dimensions of human behavior. Engel believed that the apparent crisis in American psychiatry was really a reflection of a larger crisis in American medicine, a "crisis" stemming from "adherence to a model of disease no longer adequate for the scientific tasks and social responsibilities of either medicine or psychiatry" (Engel 1977, p. 129). Engel argued for the fundamental similarities of chronic diseases like diabetes and schizophrenia and proposed that "the boundaries between health and disease . . . are diffused by cultural, social, and psychological considerations." Thus, "the physician's

basic professional knowledge and skills must span the social, psychological and biological." He saw psychiatry in 1977 as "the only clinical
discipline within medicine concerned primarily with the study of man
and the human condition" but regarded medical schools as "unreceptive
if not hostile environments" to this perspective.

Over the past 20 years, research in all of medicine (including psychiatry) has been powerfully influenced by the insights of molecular
biology. The educational message of academic psychiatry departments
has been shaped by a diagnostic system born and twice revised since the
publication of Engel's paper. The biopsychosocial model is no longer the
exclusive purview of psychiatry, primary care physicians having embraced the values associated with the model in their educational programs.[1] The problem-based learning curriculum, advocated by progressive medical educators, should be an optimal framework for teaching
Engel's model. Yet, even as the latter may have penetrated to the core
of the curriculum in some schools, more recent jeremiads deplore the
changes in the health care and academic environment that appear to pay
little attention to the biopsychosocial model: "The person with the disease, the impact of the disease on the person, the way personal characteristics modify disease presentation, and the family and the community that the patient comes from are what must engage the
practitioner" and should be the goal of undergraduate medical education.
But, "during case presentations, woe to the medical student . . . who
presents a detailed psychosocial history" because "he will be labeled a
psychosocial jock and had better plan on an internship at St. Elsewhere"
(Eisenberg 1995, p. 333).

Eisenberg also argues that the "monetarization" of medicine reduces
the encounter between doctor and patient to the perfunctory and generates attitudes and behaviors in doctors and hospitals that make any
humanistic message taught in medical school seem hypocritical. He does
not recommend abandoning the humanistic message in medical school

---

[1] In some respects, the psychiatry departments in some schools have become less
connected to the biopsychosocial model when they have focused their teaching on
diagnostic criteria and psychopharmacology. In contrast, a number of primary care
departments have enthusiastically embraced the biopsychosocial model in their educational offerings.

teaching but proposes instead a broad-gauged advocacy effort on behalf of humane values in health care (Eisenberg 1995). To the degree that medical schools choose to emphasize a biopsychosocial model in their teaching about human health and disease, the teaching programs in primary care and psychiatry will be given greater visibility in the curriculum. Unfortunately, as economic pressures build on faculty in these programs to generate income to support substantial portions of their salaries through patient care, there will be fewer incentives to teach.

Addressing the Costs of Education

In a recent article in the *New England Journal of Medicine,* Shea et al. (1996) found that the net reimbursement to the department of medicine at Columbia for teaching was $16 per hour for full-time faculty members, after the cost of fringe benefits was excluded. More than 75% of faculty teaching (excluding continuing medical education [CME] and advanced fellows) was devoted to residents. Less than one-quarter of the teaching time was devoted to medical students. Shea and colleagues acknowledged that they could not completely separate the teaching of medical students and residents because some aspects of clerkship teaching brought residents and medical students into the same learning environment.[2]

Parenthetically, the educational environment for residents impacts substantially on the education of medical students in most clerkships, because the teaching of medical students by residents strengthens both the residents' and the medical students' learning. This simultaneous learning is true of all specialties and is critical in the core clerkships

---

[2] The article by Shea et al. (1996) had serious limitations in being able to access only departmental rather than institutional data, in being unable to separate out the costs of undergraduate and graduate medical education (GME), and in offering no comparative data among departments of medicine in different medical schools or among different clinical and basic science departments within their own school. Nevertheless, it offers one published example of an effort to spell out a department of medicine's sources of funding—and it highlights the relatively small portion of support that the department receives from the medical school for teaching.

(medicine, pediatrics, psychiatry, obstetrics/gynecology, surgery, and primary care).

Table 3–1 highlights the sources of support for full-time faculty in the department of medicine at Columbia, as reported by Shea et al. (1996). Only 1.13% of the total income of the department that could be used for faculty salary support came from the medical school. The authors concluded that "uncompensated teaching time is likely to become an issue in an era in which financial compensation for physicians' activities is more closely watched" (Shea et al. 1996, p. 167). In general, as medical schools face serious limitations in their ability to shift costs from clinical income to support education (Kassirer 1994), they will need to confront the costs of their educational infrastructure and make certain that scarce educational dollars are being directed to the teaching mission.

This goal will be easier to accomplish in some locations than in others. Tuition dollars and endowments generally fail to cover the costs of undergraduate medical education (Jolin et al. 1991). Public schools in most parts of the country have experienced a relative decline in state

TABLE 3–1

Sources of salary support for full-time faculty members of the department of medicine, 1992–1993

Source	Amount ($)	Percentage of total
Clinical revenues	19,817,195	73.84
Sponsored research	2,810,040	10.47
Hospital payments for clinical activities	2,127,966	7.93
Hospital payments for teaching and administration	1,157,786	4.31
Medical school payments for teaching and administration	303,304	1.13
Gifts and endowments	620,249	2.31
Total	26,836,540	

Note. Data in this table are based on 174 of the 188 full-time faculty members for whom teaching hours were tabulated. The other 14 faculty members received no funds directly from the departmental practice plan, and three were paid directly from hospital budgets because they held administrative positions; one was paid directly from university budgets because he held an administrative position in the dean's office, and one was paid by another department, in which he held his primary appointment. The amounts shown include salary and fringe benefits.

Source. Shea et al. (1996).

support of operations. Where hospital administration is governed by an independent board of trustees, decisions about support for the combined educational infrastructure are usually beyond the purview of the dean of the medical school.[3] Within a number of universities, a significant amount of support for the infrastructure of the university comes from revenues generated by the clinical and/or research activities of the medical center. As these revenues have plateaued or begun to decline, questions are being raised by the universities regarding the financial costs of tenure in the medical schools and the resources necessary to serve the educational mission of the latter. Faculty in the medical school chafe at the dollars that flow from the medical school to the university, which means that less funding is available to support operations in the medical school. Both medical school and university administration need to confront the need for mutual accountability regarding the justification for overhead charged by the university to the medical school on the one hand and a proper accounting of the essential costs of medical education on the other.

At this juncture, too many of the hidden costs of education and research are buried within departmental budgets in the medical school. In many departments of psychiatry (as in primary care), the budget strains to support the educational costs of faculty time. In some medical schools, departmental support of faculty salaries reverts to the dean's office when the faculty member resigns or retires. However, the workload of the departing faculty member must be picked up by remaining faculty. Since psychiatry departments currently cannot generate a meaningful surplus in clinical revenue, and the chair's ability to pay faculty incentives for extra work is usually tied to the generation of surplus clinical income, there would appear to be no way to offer remaining faculty incentive to put forth the extra effort required unless the funds supporting the departing member's salary remain with the department.

In settings in which the curriculum is now centrally rather than departmentally managed, the accountability for quality and costs of teaching can be convoluted. For the most part, the centrally managed curriculum still depends on faculty resources that are under the purview

---

[3] Deans are also aware that funds sequestered in some departmental budgets are not available to support the institutional costs of education or to invest in research.

of department heads (Reynolds et al. 1995). Regardless of whether the curriculum is centrally or departmentally managed, there is a need to develop methodologies to allocate resources and rewards based on the real costs of education. The development of cost- and quality-sensitive educational initiatives should be approached with the same urgency as the clinical delivery systems are in addressing issues of cost, quality, and opportunity. In the educational area, this development should involve educational consortia, teleconferencing, and greater use of biological, behavioral, and social scientists in other parts of the university for teaching in the medical school curriculum (and vice versa). While the past two decades have been marked by educational innovations such as problem-based learning and the introduction of clinical medicine in the first two years of medical school (and the extension of basic science learning into the final two years of medical school), most educational planning and implementation efforts have not been budget driven.

The Broad Educational Mission of Academic Psychiatry

Nearly all of the respondent departments of psychiatry are involved in the education of medical students, nonpsychiatric physicians, psychiatric residents and advanced clinical and research fellows, and other mental health professionals. Some departments are also known for their efforts in the continuing education of clinicians in practice. Although some of the most prestigious psychiatry departments measure their educational success in the quality and number of resident applicants and graduates, psychiatry's role in the education of medical students, primary care physicians, and other mental health professionals, as well as in the continuing education of clinicians in practice, may be most relevant in the era of managed care. The survey data of psychiatry departments and the case studies serve to highlight the degree to which the educational mission of individual departments is differentially amplified by emphasis on 1) the advancement of knowledge through basic, clinical, and health services research; 2) the development of high-quality service programs, including programs in the public sector; and 3) the education of general physicians and other mental health care professionals.

Medical Student Teaching

Most of the respondent psychiatry departments (43 of 48) teach in all four years of the undergraduate curriculum. In the first two years of the curriculum, they may be responsible for teaching behavioral science materials relevant to health care, aspects of psychopathology and substance abuse, human development and sexuality, as well as neuroscience and psychopharmacology (Table 3–2). When medical educators today are being encouraged to teach principles of population medicine to their students, psychiatry faculty already have a rich tradition of population-based models on which to draw for information. Psychiatrists and primary care physicians play an important role in emphasizing psychosocial aspects of patient care within the integrated case materials of the problem-based curriculum. During the clinical years, psychiatry serves as one of the five or six required clerkships. As shown in Table 3–3, the clerkship in the responding departments generally runs from 4 to 8 weeks in duration.

Table 3–4 illustrates that most of the respondent department heads project significant changes in undergraduate clinical education in the next 4 years. Some departments project greater faculty involvement in preclinical teaching via problem-based learning and other interdisciplinary teaching programs, more basic science teaching in the clinical years, greater use of information technology, more elective offerings, and other changes in the curriculum. The preclinical curriculum should offer research-intensive departments of psychiatry the opportunity to highlight their expertise in neuroscience, human genetics, psychopharma-

TABLE 3-2

Medical school courses offered by 43 responding departments of psychiatry

Course	Number of departments offering course
Behavioral science	34
Introduction to the patient	18
Psychiatry	15
Neuroscience	10
Problem-based learning	9

TABLE 3-3

Length of psychiatry clerkships offered by 45 responding departments
of psychiatry

Clerkship length (weeks)	Number of departments
6	27
8	11
5	3
4	3
7	1

TABLE 3-4

Selected changes in 44 responding undergraduate psychiatric education
programs, academic year 1995–1996 to 2000–2001

Change	Number of departments
More ambulatory teaching	34
More education in primary care	24
Increased interdisciplinary teaching	12
Increased exposure to information technology, informatics	10
Curriculum changes	9
More basic science teaching in clinical years	8
More electives	7
Problem-based learning	6
Increased involvement of clinical, voluntary faculty	5
More teaching hours	4
Less lecture time in preclinical years	4
Decreased logistical and financial support for education	4
Increased emphasis on cost-effective therapy	4
Decreased specialty clerkships	4
Decreased size and length of programs	3
Structured exams	3
More emphasis on consultation and liaison	2
More student-enrichment programs	1

cology, epidemiology, developmental psychobiology, and behavioral and
social science. Through the application of interactive video technology
and computer-based learning, all departments of psychiatry should be
able to teach across a broad segment of the preclinical curriculum. The

introduction of the problem-based curriculum in the first 2 years of medical school has demonstrated the pedagogical efficacy of faculty who are able to learn and mentor well in areas of knowledge in which they are not experts. The learning environment is a collaborative one between students and teachers. The paradigm should be one in which psychiatrists are quite comfortable; indeed, in two of the case study departments, individual faculty have been leaders in curriculum reform and recipients of Teacher of the Year Awards (Colorado and Maryland).

Historically, psychiatry departments (like other specialties) have utilized the clerkship as a major recruitment vehicle to attract interested students to the specialty. Traditionally, the clerkship has emphasized the inpatient treatment of psychiatric patients, with a smattering of supervised outpatient, emergency, and medical consult activities. In the conventional inpatient clerkship experience, medical students were often given substantial responsibility in the care of patients. Patient care was not compromised because of the longer inpatient lengths of stay, as well as the collaborative style of the multidisciplinary treatment teams, on these units. Many medical students loved their psychiatry clerkship inpatient experience, which reinforced their identity as professionals. The outpatient rotations offered during the traditional psychiatry clerkship were more akin to the students' experiences on other specialty services, where their responsibility for patient care was necessarily constrained. Because managed behavioral health care has severely restricted the use of the hospital to crisis intervention and stabilization over brief lengths of stay (generally under 1 week), psychiatric education is being challenged in the same way that the traditional internal medicine clerkship has been challenged. The latter has been obliged to shift its educational programs from the inpatient unit and subspecialty clinic to ambulatory primary care practices.

As noted in Table 3–4, many chairs envision more intensive faculty involvement in ambulatory primary care and psychiatry teaching settings during required clerkships over the next 4 years. At this writing, based on the observations in most of the case study departments,[4] it is not clear that the field has learned how to incorporate the changes in the health care delivery system and the new priorities of medical education

---

[4] Dartmouth being the probable exception.

into its thinking about medical student teaching. The inpatient experience is still the core of the clerkship. Yet the vast majority of medical students will not routinely encounter in their future practices the types of acute care crises presented by mentally ill patients during inpatient stays designed to stabilize their conditions.

Medical students need to acquire the skills of history taking, lifestyle and other risk assessment, pharmacotherapy, and counseling to better serve the needs of patients seen in primary care settings. However, because the majority of patients seen in these settings do not meet criteria for Axis I disorders (see Chapter 5), the medical students would be better served by sensitive mentorship on the biopsychosocial aspects of patient care than on the details of DSM-IV (American Psychiatric Association 1994). They certainly require knowledge of the latter to pass their medical licensing examination, but the psychiatry clerkship should help to make them better (and more sensitive) physicians. The clerkship should also introduce them to the types of clinical services available to patients with psychiatric disorders, including partial hospital and intensive outpatient care; residential treatment; services to special populations such as children, the elderly, and addicted patients; and self-help groups such as Alcoholics Anonymous.

Graduate Medical Education in Psychiatry

Graduate medical education (GME) programs in psychiatry are being buffeted by a number of factors that serve to question some of the core premises of residency training in the specialty, including 1) the size of the workforce and trainee pool,[5] 2) the dual impact of managed care and new Medicare requirements on the traditional educational requirements of the residency review committee in psychiatry and the essential development of clinical autonomy among residents, and 3) the recent approval of added qualifications and postresidency fellowships in a variety of psychiatric subspecialties.

---

[5] Broadly speaking, adequate workforce issues include the decline of interest in psychiatry as a specialty among United States medical school graduates, uncertainty regarding a possible surplus of professionals in the field, and questions relating to the clinical practice boundaries between neurology, primary care, psychiatry, and other mental health professions.

The most difficult challenge facing residency training directors is the need to train a cadre of informed clinicians who are capable of changing practice patterns in response to new research findings or changes in the structure of the health care system. Many psychiatrists trained in the 1960s were strongly influenced by the predominant psychoanalytic views of treatment and were not prepared for developments in psychopharmacology or the demands of managed behavioral health care. Others received their training within large public or private psychiatric hospitals and often needed to acquire skills as outpatient clinicians after the completion of their training. These examples highlight the importance of training psychiatrists for lifelong learning and change—and not merely according to the tenets of the current fashion. At the same time, the emphasis of managed behavioral health care on reducing the costs of care and of making clinicians accountable for costs and outcome are likely to continue.

Physician Workforce Capacity: General Issues

"(E)fforts to achieve a balance of physician supply with the requirements for physician services has been a preoccupation of health planners for decades" (Tarlov 1995, p. 1558). Concern about physician shortages from the late 1950s until 1970 led to a doubling of first-year enrollment in medical schools between 1965 and 1980 and the relaxation of immigration requirements to permit international medical graduates to enter GME programs in the United States. Since the report of the Graduate Medical Education National Advisory Committee (GMENAC) in 1980, there has been a concern about physician surplus (Graduate Medical Education National Advisory Committee 1980).[6]

National projections of specialist-specific surpluses do not account for substantial regional differences in the distribution of specialist and generalist physicians (Cooper 1995). Nevertheless, a number of training programs in the surgical subspecialties were downsized or closed as a

---

[6] While the GMENAC report argued that there was danger of a surplus of many specialties, it projected a significant shortfall of general and child psychiatrists. These were deemed "shortage specialties."

consequence of a perceived surplus of professionals in the field, and medical student perceptions of physician surplus in specific specialties has impacted on the residency pool of United States medical school graduates in those specialties (Kassebaum and Szenas 1995). Two recent reports argue that physician workforce projections need to take into account the number of nonphysician clinicians in a broad array of in-dependent practices or in service as alternative service providers (e.g., nurse anesthetists) (Osterweis et al. 1996; Tarlov 1995). Many of the generic issues related to questions of physician surplus and GME capacity are relevant to psychiatry.

Workforce Issues and GME Capacity in Psychiatry

Through the 1960s and mid-1970s psychiatry enjoyed unprecedented popularity as a specialty of choice among graduating medical students, attracting as many as 8% of American medical school graduates[7] (Sierles and Taylor 1995). In some Northeastern medical schools, a substantially higher percentage of graduates chose to specialize in psychiatry during this era. In the late 1970s, the field lost some of its popularity, and the percentage of American medical school graduates choosing psychiatry dropped to 4% in 1980 (Sierles and Taylor 1995). This percentage stabilized through the 1980s, despite a 33% increase in the number of residency positions in psychiatry between 1980 and 1988[8] (Sierles and Taylor 1995). The increase in GME capacity was driven, in part, by the belief that psychiatry (and particularly child psychiatry) was a shortage specialty (Graduate Medical Education National Advisory Committee 1980).

Although the total number of positions has mostly stabilized in the past 8 years, there has been a precipitous decline in interest in psychiatry among United States medical school graduates over the past 6 years.

---

[7] A number of factors probably contributed to this trend, including National Institute of Mental Health (NIMH) support of summer fellowships for medical students, the expansion of employment opportunities for psychiatry in the public sector and in outpatient psychotherapy/psychoanalytic practice, the sense of a profound change in the care of the mentally ill that attracted the idealism of students during an idealistic time, and the promise of psychopharmacology.

[8] This increase occurred at a time when matriculation at United States medical schools had stabilized after a 15-year period of growth.

The percentage of residency slots filled by international medical school graduates has increased by 66.67% between 1990–1991 and 1994–1995 (21.5% in 1990–1991 to 35.4% in 1994–1995) (J. H. Scully, unpublished data, 1995). Moreover, only 51.5% of entering postgraduate year (PGY) I residents in psychiatry in 1994–1995 were graduates of United States medical schools (J. H. Scully, 1995).[9] While the number may increase slightly in the next few years, and some individuals may choose to transfer into psychiatry after the PGY I year, the leaders of the field need to determine whether the present trends among United States medical school graduates are reversible or will continue in the long term. If the latter manifests, it is not clear that the field can sustain the present capacity for GME, because the federal government is contemplating eliminating subsidies for GME for most international medical school graduates.[10]

---

[9] Student perception of psychiatry as a surplus specialty, a specialty with an uncertain economic future under managed behavioral health care, or a specialty with vague practice boundaries is bound to impact on psychiatry's popularity among United States medical school graduates. The humanistic emphasis in psychiatry's traditional teaching, which attracted socially committed students in the past, is now embraced by primary care training programs. Kassebaum and Szenas (1995) have noted that among 1991 medical school graduates, psychiatry was quite successful in maintaining the interest in the field that these students had at admission to medical school. Indeed, psychiatry had the highest retention rate (42.4%) of choice of specialty from matriculation to graduation. This information contrasts with data collected from 1994 graduates, where the comparable retention rate had dropped to 34%. The generalist specialties showed higher retention rates in 1994 and greater penetration among initially undecided students. The trends place psychiatry clearly among those specialties perceived to have a surplus of clinicians.

[10] At this writing the Medicare program continues to serve as the principal underwriter of the costs of graduate medical education (GME) through its support of resident salaries, or direct medical education (DME) costs, and the allocated indirect costs of their education, or indirect medical education (IME) costs. Medicare limits support for GME through the period necessary for initial specialty board eligibility, thus restricting the ability of hospitals to support fellowship training in subspecialties (including psychiatric subspecialties). Various proposals in Congress could mandate a significant decrease in Medicare support for specialty training, in an effort to increase the percentage of generalist physicians. There is also pressure to discontinue support for international medical graduates. If these efforts proceed, there could be a substantial decrease in the number of Medicare-supported residency training slots in psychiatry.

Table 3–5 lists the total number of residents presently in responding programs, the number of PGY II residents in 1995–1996 and projected 5 years, and the number of clinical and research advanced fellowships being offered in 1995–1996 and projected to 2000–2001. Given the multiple pressures affecting graduate medical education in psychiatry, the projected 15% reduction in the number of PGY II residents (by the year 2000) seems modest. Slightly more than one-third of psychiatric residency positions are offered at institutions apart from academic health centers. It is possible that more substantial reductions are planned in this sector or among academic programs that have not responded to the survey. Nevertheless, these limited data suggest that there is no consensus in the field on reducing the number of residency slots.

Would a 25%–33% reduction in GME capacity be a reasonable response to the shifting balance of international and United States medical school graduates, as well as the uncertainties of the psychiatry workforce? If a reduction in GME capacity of this magnitude is contemplated, is it more effective to reduce the size of all programs or to drop programs that are unable to meet the requirements of clinical training and didactic education in this managed care era?[11] What are the dangers of

TABLE 3-5

Number of residents, PGY II residents, clinical advanced fellows, and research fellows in 45 responding departments, academic year 1995–1996 and projection for 2000–2001

	1995–1996 academic year	2000–2001 academic year	Change (%)
Residents	1,492		
PGY II residents	374	318	(15)
Clinical advanced fellows (graduating)	204	200	(2)
Research advanced fellows (graduating)	78	84	8

[11] The merger of training programs at Sheppard-Pratt and the University of Maryland offers one model for reducing GME capacity, without the loss of a critical mass of trainees.

implementing a GME cut of this scope? What alternative educational opportunities (to GME) are currently open to academic psychiatry? The leadership of academic psychiatry and the residency review committee need to develop thoughtful answers and strategies in relation to these questions, but a substantial reduction in the number of residency slots in psychiatry seems inevitable.

Is There a Surplus of Psychiatrists?

Projections of psychiatric workforce needs depend entirely on the design and structure of the health care systems on which they are based, including questions of access to care (gatekeeper versus self-referral), the distribution of responsibilities between primary care physicians and specialists (and among mental health disciplines), the shift from inpatient to ambulatory care settings, and the method for determining the mental health benefit. If the demand for psychiatric services is based on the traditional closed staff model HMO, at least one author has projected a present surplus of 25,712 psychiatrists—the highest rate of surplus physicians among specialties in the United States (Weiner 1994). In contrast to these data, the *Journal of the American Medical Association* has reported that unemployment or underemployment for 1994 psychiatric residency graduates was extremely low (1.3%) compared with other specialties (Miller et al. 1996). These data do not suggest a current surplus. Moreover, any realistic projection of workforce needs should account for state public and forensic mental health systems and the federal Department of Veterans Affairs, which serve the chronic and severely mentally ill and addicted populations.

Workforce projections on the basis of unmet need would suggest that psychiatric practice should be a growth area. Two large-scale epidemiological surveys over the past two decades have identified relatively high rates of untreated mental illness in the community and in primary care settings (Kessler et al. 1994; Regier et al. 1988). There are also a significant number of symptomatic individuals who prefer to pay for their psychiatric care out of pocket (Klerman et al. 1992). This group accounts for a significant amount of care by mental health professionals and needs to be considered in workforce needs projections.

Apart from the issue of need, workforce projections for psychiatry must consider the skills and roles of psychiatrists that may (or may not) differentiate them from other mental health professionals, primary care physicians, and neurologists. Some have argued that psychiatry should be linked to neurology as a consultant specialty focusing on clinical neuroscience (Lieberman and Rush 1996). According to this scenario, there would appear to already be a substantial surplus of psychiatrists. There is also the perception that a significant percentage of patients with psychiatric disorders are being treated (and could be treated) by primary care physicians using newer psychotropic medications (see Chapter 5). In this model, psychosocial services could be delivered by other trained mental health professionals. Unfortunately, data on the quality of services for depressed patients by primary care physicians suggest some room for improvement (Tiemens et al. 1996).

Academic psychiatry departments, by virtue of their role in the education of the full spectrum of mental health professions (and some primary care residents) in the diagnosis, treatment, and referral of patients with mental and addictive disorders, are in a unique position to initiate a broad debate among the involved professions on the essential skills and roles in the delivery of services to mentally ill and addicted patients. Table 3–6 denotes the role of respondent departments in the education of other mental health professionals in 1995–1996 and as projected for the year 2000. No significant reductions in workforce training are planned. Currently, 10 departments of psychiatry receive funding for faculty time spent in the education of other mental health professionals.

TABLE 3-6

Number of other mental health professional students educated in psychiatry departments, academic year 1995–1996 and projection for 2000–2001

Other mental health professionals	Number of psychiatry departments	1995–1996 academic year	2000–2001 academic year
Psychology interns	28	168	159
Social work students	17	130	138
Master's degree nurses and physician assistants	8	40	48

Content Issues in GME in Psychiatry

Table 3–7 lists changes responding chairs expect to implement in their residency programs by the beginning of the century. There appears to be a consensus that training experiences must be adapted to fit a changing

TABLE 3-7

Proposed changes in graduate medical education programs reported by 45 psychiatry departments

Change	Number of responses
Provide more ambulatory care experience	25
Offer residency in primary care settings	21
Decrease number of residents	16
Increase managed care training	16
Implement joint residency programs	13
Emphasize brief therapies	9
Offer more advanced fellowships	9
Offer longitudinal experiences in integrated systems	9
Provide more experience with computers and information technology	7
Provide more research training	7
Encounter financial and administrative problems	7
Other	7
Develop comprehensive community training sites	6
Decrease dependence on residents for clinical service	5
Offer UR/QA electives for all residents	4
Create more part-time training opportunities	4
Develop a Firm Model	4
Require reading lists and exams	3
Develop regional consortia for teaching	2
Merge programs	2
Offer more use of residents to teach medical students	2
Provide more tertiary care consultation experience	1
Include fewer affiliated sites	1
Reduce research time	1
Increase work with physician extenders	1
Create new teaching track	1
Provide better links with basic social sciences	1
Increase substance abuse experience	1
Increase dependence on voluntary faculty	1
Develop comprehensive public psychiatry training	1

clinical environment. Because of managed behavioral health care, patients' responses to pharmacological and psychosocial-behavioral treatments now occur in alternative venues to traditional inpatient care. Inpatient rotations no longer provide residents with the opportunity to get to know patients through episodes of illness and recovery, to develop a therapeutic relationship, or to learn the effects of sequential treatment interventions over time. Of the responding chairs, 20% highlighted the importance of offering residents the opportunity to follow patients longitudinally across a range of treatment venues, but less than 10% specifically referred to the implementation of a "Firm Model." The latter was developed as a model of residency training in Britain and involves the assignment of the trainee to a practitioner (or clinical delivery team) with longitudinal responsibility for population-based health care. One application of the model to psychiatry is highlighted in the case report from Dartmouth Medical School. If the training program at Dartmouth is representative of the future residency training experience, there will be less emphasis on fixed clinical rotations and greater emphasis on the broad range of clinical skills necessary for the longitudinal care of patients across all venues of care.

Meyer and Sotsky (1995, p. 74) suggested that the residency review committee in psychiatry focus on "the . . . capacity of training programs to prepare residents for work in managed care settings" and consult in primary care ambulatory settings, as well as the traditional tertiary care medical-surgical unit. They urged "training in administrative psychiatry with special reference to managed care issues, . . . the organization and financing of mental health services, utilization and clinical management, and clinical ethics. For chronically ill patients, residents need to learn new models based upon principles of psychosocial rehabilitation . . . , a thorough grounding in medication management, including patients being treated by non-medical mental health clinicians. Psychotherapy training [should include] a variety of brief individual, family and group psychotherapies," as well as some long-term therapy because some patients will continue to need and be willing to pay for this modality.

The medical director of one of the larger behavioral health companies (W. Goldman, personal communication, February 1996) agreed with the preceding skills list but added that residency graduates also should have excellent facility with electronic information exchange, the capacity to recognize and treat dual mental illness and addictive disorders, and competence in the diagnosis and treatment of the basic medical care needs of the chronically and persistently mentally ill. Goldman believes that graduates must learn to accept responsibility for patient outcomes and that residency training should do a better job of integrating pharmacotherapy and psychotherapy skills. Training should emphasize diagnosis and treatment in ambulatory settings.

Some of the changes in residency education projected by the responding departments focused on skills and roles, while others focused on changes in the process of education. Tables 3–8 and 3–9 list the essential skills and future roles of psychiatrists as noted by the department chairs. The skills and roles required by the future psychiatrist, as projected by the responding department heads, seem consistent with the direction of managed behavioral health care.

TABLE 3-8

Essential skills for psychiatrists reported by 34 departments

Skill	Number of responses
Medical consultation	23
Supervision of other mental health personnel	21
Medication management	17
Diagnosis and evaluation	16
Working in health professional teams	9
Other (includes general psychotherapy)	7
Brief psychotherapy	6
Therapy for special populations (e.g., substance abuse)	3
Group psychotherapy	3
Case management	3
Population-based practice	2
Knowledge of information technology	2
Family therapy	1

TABLE 3-9

Future role of psychiatrists reported by 32 departments

Role	Number of responses
Specialist/Consultant	30
Other (includes administrative roles)	19
Practice	13
Teaching and clinical training	12
Research	9
Primary care for the chronically mentally ill	6
Managed care positions	5
Public-sector positions	3

The Impact of Managed Care and Medicare Regulations on Residency Training

The residency review committee and individual programs are being challenged to implement or accommodate significant changes in emphasis and content over a relatively brief period of time. Managed behavioral health programs and new Medicare regulations are forcing academic psychiatry departments to rethink and reconfigure their GME programs. It is unclear whether programs will be permitted to grant residents sufficient practice autonomy (under supervision) to enable them to mature as clinicians. At Sheppard-Pratt, residents are not prevented from providing services under contracts with some managed behavioral health care companies but are excluded by others. At Colorado, the managed care unit does not offer training experiences for residents or medical students. While at least one managed behavioral health care company (GreenSpring) funds advanced fellowship training in managed behavioral health care at the University of Maryland and the University of Medicine and Dentistry of New Jersey (Newark), the real challenge to these companies and to training programs will be the inculcation of high-quality, cost-sensitive practice patterns within general residency training programs. To mature as clinicians, psychiatric residents need to experience the richness of the doctor-patient relationship as full participants during their training.

This issue also seems not to have been recognized in the formulation of recent Medicare regulations (Federal Register 1995), which are impacting on the *process* of psychiatric residency education, in the relationship between trainees, patients, and faculty. The language in the regulations suggests greater sensitivity to the training needs in the primary care disciplines than in psychiatry: "we recognized that application of this policy to the reimbursement of teaching physicians in family practice residency programs raised special concerns about the viability of these programs. . . . While teaching physicians supervise . . . care [given by family practice residents], a general requirement that teaching physicians be physically present during all visits to the family practice center would *undermine the development of the physician/patient relationship . . . [and] would be incompatible with the way family practice centers are organized and staffed* [italics mine]" (Federal Register 1995, p. 63140). "In light of the comments, we have concluded that an exception should not be limited to family practice programs. . . . We believe that the types of GME programs most likely to qualify for this exception include: family practice and some programs in general internal medicine, geriatrics and pediatrics." Under the exception, a teaching physician may supervise up to four residents at any given time and "have no other responsibilities." The supervisory function does not require that the faculty member and the patient also establish a relationship (Federal Register 1995, p. 63146). In contrast, for psychiatric residencies, "the teaching physician may observe a resident's treatment of patients only through one-way mirrors or video equipment" and must meet "with the patient after the visit" (Federal Register 1995, p. 63147).

The pattern now established by Medicare is likely to be followed by other payers. The new Medicare rules seem quite sensitive to the requirements of teaching and trainee autonomy development in primary care practices. In contrast, they increase the teaching costs (one faculty member per resident) and complicate the doctor-patient relationship in psychiatry. The new rules will certainly challenge departments and the residency review committee to review the process of clinical education in the specialty.

Subspecialty Training in Psychiatry

Apart from child psychiatry, which has been a distinct subspecialty for many years, psychiatry had not developed clear subspecialty areas of clinical practice and advanced training until recently. Starting in the late 1980s added qualifications were sought for geriatric psychiatry, addiction psychiatry, forensic psychiatry, and consultation-liaison psychiatry. Table 3–10 describes the enrollment progression from academic year 1991–1992 to academic year 1994–1995 in child psychiatry, geriatric psychiatry, addiction psychiatry, forensic psychiatry, and consultation-liaison psychiatry across the United States. Data are also offered for advanced research and psychotherapy fellowships. The data suggest a dramatic decline in the number of fellows in addiction psychiatry programs, which should be of concern to advocates of subspecialty training in this field. Child psychiatry has experienced substantial growth during this period, but other areas of specialization have not experienced similar increases. Given these data, and the lack of substantial stipend or educational support for fellowship training beyond board eligibility, the future of the psychiatric subspecialties may come into question. Yet among the respondent department chairs, little change was projected for the year 2000 in the number of graduating advanced clinical fellows (Table 3–6). Reductions projected in child psychiatry were offset by increases in geriatric, forensic, and consultation-liaison psychiatry graduates. An 8% increase in the number of graduating research fellows was projected (Table 3–6).

As described previously, at least one of the leaders of the managed behavioral health industry (W. Goldman, personal communication, February 1996) argues for broadly skilled psychiatrists who can diagnose and treat comorbid addictive disorders. The future health system will need psychiatrists who can serve as consultants in adult or pediatric health care settings and who can offer direct services to adult or pediatric patients with mental or addictive disorders. Should residency training in adult and child psychiatry prepare graduates for all of these potential roles, without the need for additional subspecialty training? In the world of managed behavioral and general health care, is it better to be a broadly trained general psychiatrist or a subspecialist in addiction, geriatric, or consultation-liaison psychiatry?

TABLE 3-10

Enrollment in psychiatry programs by type, academic years 1990–1991 through 1994–1995

Program type	1990–1991		1991–1992		1992–1993		1993–1994		1994–1995	
	Number enrolled	Percentage	Number enrolled	Percentage	Number enrolled	Percentage	Number enrolled	Percentage	Number enrolled	Percentage
General psychiatry	5,069	84.3	5,081	82.5	5,088	83.5	5,129	84.6	5,121	84.1
Combined general and child psychiatry	155	2.6	268	4.4	199	3.3	n/a		n/a	
Child psychiatry	494	8.2	563	9.1	584	9.6	679	11.2	754	12.4
Research	n/a*		58	0.9	75	1.2	59	1.0	56	0.9
Geriatrics	n/a		26	0.4	32	0.5	41	0.7	36	0.6
Forensics	n/a		17	0.3	22	0.4	22	0.4	18	0.3
Consult-liaison psychiatry	n/a		25	0.4	25	0.4	18	0.3	19	0.3
Alcohol or substance abuse	n/a		22	0.4	20	0.3	17	0.3	7	0.1
Psychotherapy	n/a		3	<0.1	6	0.1	8	0.1	4	0.1
Other	298	4.9	96	1.6	44	0.7	86	1.4	74	1.2
Total	6,016	100.0	6,159	100.0	6,095	100.0	6,059	100.0	6,089	100.0

*n/a = not available

Source.   American Psychiatric Association (1996).

Subspecialization in psychiatry has had a different history than its counterparts in medicine, pediatrics, obstetrics, and surgery. Unlike the development of subspecialization in internal medicine and pediatrics, it has not been strongly linked to research, although that connection is possible. Unlike internal medicine, pediatrics, obstetrics and gynecology, or surgery, it has not been fueled by dramatically new diagnostic or therapeutic technologies with potentially higher rates of reimbursement. Subspecialties in these disciplines came during a period in which specialized areas of knowledge in medicine were valued. The psychiatric subspecialties have come of age during a time that places higher value on generalist skills. In light of all of these issues, professionals in the field need to step back and consider the place of the content of the subspecialties in relation to the general and child psychiatry curriculum. The future of most of the subspecialties in psychiatry may not yet be apparent, but the issues have changed substantially since the approval of added qualifications in each of them. There may still be an opportunity to link the development of advanced research and practice skills in some of the subspecialties in ways that will strengthen the subspecialty and psychiatry as a whole. This issue could be developed with leaders in the Department of Veterans Affairs (Chapter 6) and the relevant institutes at the National Institutes of Health (NIH).

Other Educational Issues

None of the respondent departments in the national survey or the case study departments reported that they had embarked on a strategy to link continuing education to potential network development or the opportunities in managed behavioral health care. Yet one of the leaders of the managed behavioral health industry (W. Goldman, personal communication, February 1996) has recently emphasized the opportunities: "continuing education for the existing workforce remains a neglected and unappreciated mission in academic psychiatry," and "efforts to retrain faculty are almost non-existent." If Goldman is correct, the reeducation of the existing workforce represents an important challenge and opportunity for academic psychiatry that might bring the interests of the academicians and the behavioral health companies into alignment.

The potential linkage of workforce reeducation and quality assurance and utilization review, within university-associated network providers in the community, would appear to be an excellent opportunity. The challenge to departments of psychiatry will start with the reeducation of full-time faculty.

"Current faculty may not be equipped by background, level and nature of skills or inclination to present new material competently. . . . Changing the behavior of professionals is always a daunting task . . . *with* . . . numerous studies demonstrating how difficult it is to get physicians to adopt new forms of treatment. . . . The 'trainer of the trainers' will have to understand the sociology and psychology of groups based on shared values and economic advantage, and the problems of altering the positions of such groups" (C. Van Dyke and H. J. Schlesinger, unpublished observations, August 1996). For faculty to become effective teachers of skills and roles appropriate to managed behavioral health care, they will have to acquire some new skills and knowledge. These relate principally to briefer psychotherapies, alternatives to inpatient treatment of major mental illness, the integration of psychotherapy and pharmacotherapy, and the diagnosis and treatment of patients with comorbid addictive and mental disorders. They also will need to develop attitudes that embrace responsibility and accountability for clinical outcomes and for the health and well-being of populations.

The attitudinal issues will be more difficult to address than the simple transmission of new skills and knowledge. While economic considerations affect practice patterns, it is more difficult to inculcate new skills and knowledge if physicians believe that current practice is better for the patient, more humane, technologically more challenging, more likely to achieve a long-standing better outcome, or reflective of real caring for the patient and her or his family. Practice patterns and the curriculum in psychiatry have been difficult to change because of attitudes supporting the view that long-term psychotherapy is more humane, methodologically more challenging, more likely to achieve a better long-term outcome, more reflective of real caring for the patient, and intellectually more interesting than the alternatives. The problem was not principally a deficit in skills and knowledge but attitudinal—and buttressed by a peer-reinforced system of values.

Summary

Economic pressures are focusing attention. Like the "new day" for general internists, population-based advocates in psychiatry have gained the upper hand through economic realities. But if advocates of managed behavioral health care are to avoid missing the types of opportunities that were offered to the community psychiatrists of the 1960s and 1970s, they will need to join with academic psychiatrists to develop a credible intellectual base that will inform clinical practice, identify meaningful roles and skills for *each* of the mental health disciplines within the interdisciplinary team construct, advocate and implement models of patient care that are sensitive to the functional needs of patients and families with chronic and severe mental and addictive disorders, and advance a knowledge- and skill-based professionalism capable of evolving in response to scientific understanding. Advocates of managed behavioral health are too easily caricatured as clinically naive or ill-informed and driven by an economic agenda, much as the community psychiatrists of a generation ago were characterized relative to their clinical skills and their alleged political motivations.

For faculty to help to change the way psychiatry is taught and practiced, the future roles and skills of psychiatrists should be defined in the context of both behavioral and general health care. A paradigm more comprehensive than traditional psychoanalytic perspectives, which have still not incorporated the insights of psychopharmacology into their canon after 40 years, is needed. Psychiatric practice is more than prescription writing, and psychiatric patients are more than the sum of the number of defining criteria of their disorders. Psychiatry at the millennium includes elements of primary care and psychiatry; recent advances in molecular and cellular neurobiology and other areas of basic research; clinical investigation; behavioral, psychosocial, and epidemiological research; intuitive skills; humane values; and an economically driven focus on maintaining the health of populations through something called managed behavioral health care. As voiced by Eisenberg (1995), the challenge to academic psychiatry (as to the rest of medicine) will be to strengthen its commitment to the humane values of a true biopsychosocial model and to learn how to practice and to teach it within a price-sensitive, market-driven economy and culture.

References

American Psychiatric Association: Diagnostic and Statistical Manual of Mental Disorders, 4th Edition. Washington, DC, American Psychiatric Association, 1994

Cooper RA: Perspectives on the physician workforce to the year 2020. JAMA 274:1534–1543, 1995

Eisenberg L: Medicine—molecular, monetary or more than both? JAMA 274:331–334, 1995

Engel GL: The need for a new medical model: a challenge for biomedicine. Science 196:129–135, 1977

Federal Register 60:63135–63148, 1995

Graduate Medical Education National Advisory Committee: Report of the Graduate Medical Education Advisory Committee to the Secretary, Department of Health and Human Services, Volume 1. Washington, DC, U.S. Department of Health and Human Services, 1980

Jolin LD, Jolly P, Krakower JY, et al: US medical school finances. JAMA 266:985–990, 1991

Kassebaum DG, Szenas PL: Medical students' career indecision and specialty rejection: roads not taken. Acad Med 70:937–943, 1995

Kassirer JP: Academic medical centers under siege. N Engl J Med 331:1370–1371, 1994

Kessler RC, McGonagle KA, Zhao S, et al: Lifetime and 12-month prevalence of DSM-III R psychiatric disorders in the United States: results from the National Comorbidity Survey. Arch Gen Psychiatry 51:8–19, 1994

Klerman GL, Olfson M, Leon AC, et al: Measuring the need for mental health care. Health Affairs 11:23–33, 1992

Lieberman JA, Rush AJ: Redefining the role of psychiatry in medicine. Am J Psychiatry 153:1388–1397, 1996

Meyer RE, Sotsky SM: Managed care and the role and training of psychiatrists. Health Affairs 14:65–77, 1995

Miller RS, Jonas HS, Whitcomb ME: The initial employment status of physicians completing training in 1994. JAMA 275:708–712, 1996

Osterweis M, McLaughlin CJ, Manasse HR, et al: The US Health Workforce: Power, Politics and Policy. Washington, DC, Association of Academic Health Centers, 1996

Pew Health Professions Commission: Critical Challenges: Revitalizing the Health Professions for the Twenty-First Century. Philadelphia, PA, Pew Health Professions Commission, 1995

Regier DA, Boyd JH, Burke JD Jr, et al: One-month prevalence of mental disorders in the United States. Arch Gen Psychiatry 45:977–986, 1988

Reynolds CF, Adler S, Kanter SL, et al: The undergraduate medical curriculum: centralized versus departmentalized. Acad Med 70:671–683, 1995

Shea S, Nickerson KG, Tenenbaum J, et al: Compensation to a department of medicine and its faculty members for the teaching of medical students and house staff. N Engl J Med 334:162–168, 1996

Sierles FS, Taylor MA: Decline of US medical student career choice of psychiatry and what to do about it. Am J Psychiatry 152:1416–1426, 1995

Tarlov AR: Estimating physician workforce requirements: the devil is in the assumptions. JAMA 274:1558–1560, 1995

Tiemens BG, Ormel J, Simon GE: Occurrence, recognition and outcome of psychological disorders in primary care. Am J Psychiatry 153:636–644, 1996

Weiner JP: Forecasting the effects of health reform on US physician workforce requirement: evidence from HMO staffing patterns. JAMA 272:222–230, 1994

CHAPTER 4

The Place of Research in the Mission of Academic Psychiatry

Roger E. Meyer, M.D., and Christopher J. McLaughlin

The extraordinary burgeoning of psychiatric research within American medical schools over the past 15 years may not be generally known within academic medicine. As documented by the office of research of the American Psychiatric Association (based on data provided by the National Institutes of Health [NIH]), between 1984 and 1993, NIH (formerly Alcohol, Drug Abuse and Mental Health Association [ADAMHA]) support to departments of psychiatry rose from $82.5 million (10th place among medical school departments) to $300.9 million (second place among medical school departments). This trend was associated with a number of developments that need to be highlighted. It is probably the confluence of these developments that accounts for the recent trends in research support in psychiatry. Parenthetically, even at present levels of support, the percentage of research support on psychiatric and addictive disorders relative to their prevalence in the general population and their costs to the economy is still substantially less than the comparable percentage of research support relative to the prevalence and costs of many major medical disorders.

Changes in Federal Support for Research

In the mid-1960s, the National Institute of Mental Health (NIMH) was separated from the rest of NIH and given a very broad mission to fund services to mentally ill and addicted patients,[1] training for mental health professionals, and research. Federal interest in the community-based focus of the mission peaked during the Carter administration and was abruptly terminated in 1981 when the categorical support for services administered by NIMH, National Institute on Alcohol Abuse and Alcoholism (NIAAA), and National Institute on Drug Abuse (NIDA) was transferred to a block grant. At that time, the Reagan Administration changed the mission of the three institutes of ADAMHA to emphasize research on alcoholism, drug abuse, and major mental illness and to downplay support for social research and for local service programs for mentally ill and addicted patients.

The evolutionary change in mission of these institutes was continued in 1992, when Congress authorized their transfer back to the NIH to focus exclusively on research and research training. Their service-related functions were transferred to a new agency, the Substance Abuse and Mental Health Services Administration (SAMHSA). NIMH, NIDA, and NIAAA continue to offer a very broad research portfolio that includes molecular, cellular, and behavioral neurobiology; cognitive neuroscience; human and molecular genetics; animal and human behavioral studies; functional brain imaging; clinical, prevention, and treatment research; epidemiology and psychosocial research; and health services research. It should be self-evident that the final test regarding the wisdom of the most recent reorganization will be the continuing vitality of this broad research portfolio. Yet there is a palpable feeling of anxiety within the broader research community supported by NIAAA, NIDA, and NIMH whenever some (alleged) quote about the need to consolidate neuroscience research (and to emphasize molecular neurobiology as the principal research portfolio) is attributed to unnamed leadership at NIH or the dean of a prominent medical school.

Molecular biology and molecular genetics are most likely to advance

---

[1] Initially through the construction and staffing of a nationwide system of community mental health centers.

our understanding of human diseases where the phenotypic disorder or disorders are well described, if there is strong evidence of familial transmission, and if there are relevant animal models of the human disorders. At this juncture, much needs to be done across the span of clinical and basic research to better describe the phenotypes of psychiatric disorders in the context of our growing knowledge of developmental and cognitive neuroscience to move beyond our present system of consensus-derived descriptive syndromes. The continued growth of research support within the former ADAMHA institutes is now tied more closely to the rate of growth of the NIH budget. The fate of the intramural and extramural research activities related to mental and addictive disorders within NIH has now become more dependent on attitudes toward this mission-based research agenda within the parent agency.

Other Developments Supporting the Expansion of Psychiatric Research

The emphasis on federal support for research on mental and addictive disorders since 1981 has been compatible with a number of other trends. Commencing in the late 1970s, NIMH, NIDA, and NIAAA have collaborated in the support of two major epidemiological surveys on the prevalence of mental and addictive disorders, using criteria with high reliability. These criteria were advanced by an international effort to standardize definitions of psychiatric and addictive disorders and by the efforts of the American Psychiatric Association (APA) to improve diagnostic reliability relative to these disorders in the United States. Over the past 15 years, the overall program has brought together a number of distinguished psychiatric epidemiologists, with the support of the ADAMHA, World Health Organization (WHO), and APA.

The Epidemiological Catchment Area survey of adults age 18 and over conducted between 1981 and 1985 documented a 1-year incidence of mental and addictive disorders of 22% (Regier et al. 1988). The National Comorbidity Study of 8,000 individuals aged 15 to 54 was conducted between 1990 and 1992 and documented a 1-year incidence rate of 30%, with a lifetime prevalence rate of 48% (Kessler et al. 1994). For the first time in the modern history of psychiatric epidemiology, the survey data reported incidence and prevalence of disorders rather than symptoms. The resurgence of psychiatric nosology helped to stimulate a number of other activities, including 1) disorder-specific clinical investigations; 2) industry-supported clinical trials; 3) the application of new technologies to studies of psychiatric disorders; and 4) the interests of citizen-advocacy organizations and health policy analysts in the costs of these disorders to society and the opportunities for research, prevention, and treatment. While future basic and clinical research will likely alter the present diagnostic schema, the latter has helped to shape a research agenda, as well as psychiatric practice and teaching.

In the early 1980s the Institute of Medicine (IOM) issued several reports highlighting the research opportunities on mental and addictive disorders and on alcoholism in particular (Institute of Medicine 1980; 1984; 1985). More recent IOM reports have highlighted specific opportunities in child psychiatry and addiction research, along with treatment and prevention research, brain imaging, molecular and cellular neurobiology, human genetics, and developmental and cognitive psychology (Institute of Medicine 1987; 1989a,b; 1996). The research opportunities were also highlighted by the designation of the present decade as "The Decade of the Brain" by former president Bush and both houses of Congress, as well as a number of foreign leaders.

As is well understood in our nation's capital, federal funding for a category of biomedical research does not always correlate with level of need or the breadth of scientific opportunity. The process is advanced by citizen-advocacy organizations. In the area of mental illness, citizen advocacy came of age in the 1980s, with families of the mentally ill represented by the National Alliance for the Mentally Ill (NAMI) and patients represented by such organizations as the National Depressive and Manic Depressive Association and the Anxiety Disorders Association of America. Each of these organizations (joined by the National Mental Health Association [NMHA] and several disorder-specific groups) made support for research on major mental illness a high priority of its advocacy efforts.

The linkage of citizen advocacy to support for research also helped to destigmatize mental illness for patients and families. The single most direct impact of citizen advocacy on the growth of psychiatric research since the mid-1980s has been the growth of the National Association for Research on Schizophrenia and Affective Disorders (NARSAD).

NARSAD brought together the extraordinary talents of the concerned parents of a schizophrenic adult (Connie and Steve Lieber) and Dr. Herbert Pardes (the former director of NIMH, and chair of psychiatry and dean at Columbia). The organization has focused its support on attracting young investigators, minimizing its administrative costs, and developing a model partnership between citizen advocacy and the scientific community. In the past 9 years, NARSAD has been able to award $43 million, based on the recommendations of its scientific council. It is the single greatest source of support for psychiatric researchers after NIH and industry.[2]

Within American psychiatry, the 1980s were marked by a shift in leadership in a number of academic departments to a new generation of department chairs, who placed a high priority on the development of significant research programs. Indeed, some of the leading basic scientists in neurobiology hold primary academic appointments in psychiatry departments. The APA established an office of research headed by a former official from NIMH, whose background as a psychiatrist with a strong interest in science and public policy has made the APA a strong and effective partner in advocating for psychiatric research.

Factors Associated With Research Intensity

To gain a clearer perspective on the factors associated with the rapid development of psychiatric research over the past 10 to 15 years, we secured data from NIH on research support to all psychiatry departments and medical schools for fiscal year (FY) 1994. We also devoted specific questions relative to research in the department (and research infrastructure in the medical school) in the department chairs' survey (45 respondents to this question) and solicited additional input from some of the chairs of the most successful research departments. Finally, we secured additional data and subjective impressions in some of the case reports.

In FY 1994, 48 departments of psychiatry received more than $1.0 million in grant support for research from NIH. These data are especially

---

[2] The Stanley Foundation and the MacArthur Foundation have also contributed generously to support research on mental illness.

interesting in light of the 1989 survey conducted by the APA's office of research, which found that half of the researchers in departments of psychiatry were located in the top 15 (in research support) of 116 responding departments (Pincus et al. 1993). To be defined as a researcher in that APA survey, a faculty member had to meet the following criteria: 1) spends at least 20% of time in research, 2) has authored or coauthored at least one original research article in the previous 2 years, and 3) has assigned research space or was the recipient of external funding. Only 25.8% of responding psychiatrists met criteria as researchers, and only 15% were able to spend more than 50% of their time in research. In an earlier paper by Levey et al., nearly 42% of academic internists were classified as researchers according to criteria similar to those employed in the APA survey (Levey et al. 1988). Academic psychiatry has been less effective than academic internal medicine in building an infrastructure that will support faculty devoting a substantial percentage of time to research. This discrepancy makes the recent burgeoning of psychiatric research even more remarkable. In addition, psychiatry departments have been much less successful than their counterparts in neurology or internal medicine in attracting support from NIH grant–supported M.D.–Ph.D. programs.[3] Graduates of these dual-degree programs will likely be disproportionately represented in the next generation of physician scientists.

Based on the FY 1994 data from NIH, there appears to be a strong relationship between the research ranking of a department of psychiatry in one of the top quartiles (or bottom half) and the ranking of the parent medical school. Among the 31 departments of psychiatry in the top quartile of NIH support, 21 departments were from medical schools in the top quartile, 7 were from medical schools in the second quartile, and 3 were from medical schools in the bottom half of the rankings list. Of the 62 departments of psychiatry[4] in the bottom half of the NIH

---

[3] According to data supplied by the Office of Research of the American Psychiatric Association.

[4] For this analysis, the merged departments of psychiatry at the University of Nebraska and Creighton were counted as a single department. In addition, where available, the research support coming to a principal-affiliated teaching hospital was combined with the amount of NIH support credited to the department of psychiatry

rankings, 49 were from medical schools in the bottom half, 10 were from schools in the second quartile, and 4 were from schools in the top quartile ($N = 63$ medical schools). For this 1 year of data on NIH support, 20 departments of psychiatry appeared to be doing better in NIH ranking than their parent medical schools ("overachievers") and 20 departments were ranked as relative "underachievers." Although 1 year of data does not constitute a definitive pattern, it does have face validity. We also examined other factors that might be associated with NIH research ranking, including the research infrastructure available to departments of psychiatry that responded to the survey, the presence of a public sector–academic relationship supporting research, and/or the development of niche areas of research excellence. In the next few years, intensity of managed behavioral health care penetration could affect the growth of research support in psychiatry departments.

Moy et al. recently examined the relationship between the rate of growth of NIH research support to United States medical schools across different managed care markets between 1986 and 1995 (E. Moy, A. J. Mazzaschi, R. J. Levin et al., unpublished observations, 1997). They found that between 1990 and 1995, medical schools in more intensive managed care markets experienced slower growth in the dollar amounts and numbers of NIH awards compared with schools in markets with low or medium managed care penetration. Much of this relative deficit could be explained by the slower growth of investigator-initiated (R01) awards to clinical departments in schools in high managed care markets.

Table 4–1 contrasts the research infrastructure available to departments of psychiatry in the top and second quartile of research support, compared with departments in the bottom half of NIH research support. These data were collected from among the 45 departments responding to this survey question, thus excluding data from some departments listed in the NIH data. The availability of a general clinical research

at the university (e.g., the funds for the New York State Psychiatric Institute and Columbia University's departments of psychiatry could be summed in the available NIH data; similarly, the data from McLean Hospital and Harvard's departments of psychiatry could be summed, but separate grants to the other hospital-based psychiatry programs at Harvard could not be identified in this calculation).

TABLE 4-1

Research infrastructure present in psychiatry departments by research
ranking of department

Resource present in department	Top quartile ranking (N = 11)	Second quartile ranking (N = 12)	Bottom half ranking (N = 22)
CRC	100%	58%	50%
Positron-electron tomography	64%	50%	41%
Single photon emission computed tomography	45%	58%	32%
Human genetics	82%	58%	59%
Basic neurosciences	100%	100%	82%
Health services research	91%	100%	73%
Biostatistics	91%	100%	82%
Epidemiology	82%	100%	59%
Behavioral social science	82%	83%	82%

Note. Collaborative agreements not included.

center (GCRC) and a human genetics research program almost defines
the top quartile of research-intensive departments. They are probably
also linked to the research intensity of the parent medical school. The
growing importance of functional brain imaging to clinical investigation
in psychiatry may eventually become a critical threshold for research
intensity, but at this juncture a substantial percentage of research-intensive departments do not have access to positron-emission tomography
(PET) or single photon emission computed tomography (SPECT) scan-
ning at their medical center. Some of the resources listed in Table 4–1
are institutional resources, where access by psychiatric researchers may
not be optimal (e.g., basic neuroscience research in some schools).

In the future, as individual clinical departments become less able to
fund their own essential research infrastructure, medical schools will
need to develop institution-wide collaborative efforts to assure access
to cutting-edge technology relevant to research on clinical disorders. In
this regard, research in psychiatry may be linked to other efforts in
clinical and basic neuroscience, human genetics, health services research,
clinical trials, and treatment and prevention research relative to general
and mental health issues. Dr. Herbert Pardes's description of the insti-

tutional development of a clinical trials program at Columbia is instructive (personal communication, May 1996).

"We found that clinical trials were formidable to do at Columbia in the early '90's." Industry did not appreciate the multitude of university committees that had to be traversed before one could commence a clinical trial. "We set up a special office" directed by someone knowledgeable about working with industry, and "the hospital and medical school (pooled) some of the indirect costs money . . . (from) the trials and put it at the disposal of a faculty committee (to) advise the hospital President and medical school Dean as to areas of clinical research infrastructure needing support." Columbia started a program of $50,000 starter grants for young clinical investigators (10 per year), and it has increased its clinical trials efforts eight- to ninefold. The whole process "reenergized the tumor board, clinical pharmacy, (and) imaging programs from some of the resulting monies." The school also rebuilt its clinical research center facility. Addressing research infrastructure issues from an institutional perspective in this way benefited clinical investigators in all departments. With the perception that clinical research will be adversely affected by the impact of managed care in the context of payment denials, competitive market pressures, and limited access to research subjects (Mechanic and Dobson 1996), institutional initiatives like the one described by Dr. Pardes will be critical to protect and advance clinical research across all academic departments. Between 1989 and 1993, the use of academic investigators in industry-sponsored research trials fell from 82% to 68% (Burnett 1996). This trend toward increased use of nonacademic sites for clinical trials, if continued, would be devastating to clinical research at many academic medical centers. It underlies the importance of efforts like that at Columbia to consolidate and simplify the oversight for these studies within academic centers.

Five of the top-ten-ranked departments of psychiatry (University of Pittsburgh, Yale, University of California–San Francisco,[5] University of Colorado, and Columbia University) continue to receive some core aca-

---

[5] Funds that once came to this department to support education, research, and indigent patient care through the state department of mental health were transferred to the department of higher education to support psychiatry programs at UCSF/ Langley Porter.

demic support that has historically been linked to the public sector. The University of Pennsylvania and the University of California at San Diego have benefited from close linkages with local Department of Veterans Affairs hospitals. Several other relatively highly ranked research programs, including the Medical College of Pennsylvania (Allegheny), the University of Michigan, Harvard (Massachusetts Mental Health Center), New York University (Nathan Kline Research Center), the University of Maryland, the University of Iowa, and the University of California–Los Angeles, benefit from direct or indirect public-sector support for research. The importance of public service–academic linkages to research are highlighted in the case reports from Maryland, Dartmouth, and Colorado.

According to a 1987–1988 survey by the APA's office of research, 57% of the states support some research on mental illness, and 29% support some research on substance abuse (Pincus and Fine 1992). In aggregate, such state support represented 0.3% of total state expenditures for mental health. While the total would appear to be rather small, it is not clear whether this level of effort has been maintained since 1988. For academic psychiatry in a number of centers of excellence, this state support has been critical. Although some academic clinical disciplines historically have been able to shift costs for support for faculty research time from surplus clinical income, this option has been difficult to implement in psychiatry because of the nature of psychiatric practice. (Under managed behavioral health care, it is now impossible to shift costs in this way since there is no surplus clinical income.)

In some respects, public-sector support has helped academic psychiatry in ways that surplus clinical income has helped other academic clinical disciplines to develop a research infrastructure. As described by Dr. Herbert Pardes, "the world class status" of the state-funded New York State Psychiatric Institute at Columbia has been a major factor in the academic and research success of this department, but its ongoing success is subject to the uncertainties of state budgets and politics (personal communication, May 1996). Because these programs are so critical to the future research mission of academic psychiatry, the leaders of academic health centers (AHCs) and psychiatry department chairs need to work together with local citizen-advocacy organizations and leaders of public-sector programs to develop mechanisms to protect these programs from downsizing or closure. In the past decade, separate threats have been experienced by major state-funded psychiatric research programs in New York, Maryland, Massachusetts, Illinois, and Michigan (Wayne State). Given the small size of the effort relative to the overall mental health budgets of these states, and given the importance of state support of research to the viability of the research enterprise, it is critical to develop funding models that can shield these programs from the often unintended consequences of the actions of legislative budget cutters or new political leaders.

In addition to the relationship between research rank of the psychiatry department and research rank of medical school, as well as that between the availability of public-sector funding and research productivity, we also looked more closely at some of the departments that had been able to develop research resources that placed them at a higher rank than would be expected from the ranking of their medical school and some innovative efforts that have been developed to support the research infrastructure in psychiatry. Where academic departments of psychiatry do not have an adequate infrastructure to support clinical, basic, and health services research, they have sometimes turned to innovative regional collaborative arrangements.

One such arrangement, the Chicago Consortium for Psychiatric Research, was launched in 1986 in response to the threatened downsizing (or closure) of the research programs at the Illinois State Psychiatric Institute (ISPI) (B. M. Astrachan, R. A. deVito, M. A. Andriukaitis, personal communication, May 1996). Following a successful effort to block the effort, the chairs of all psychiatry departments in Chicago (and the research director of ISPI) secured a planning grant from the Chicago Community Trust to develop a structure to foster psychiatric research across all of the academic departments (and ISPI) in a collaborative and coordinated manner. The resulting consortium applied for and received nearly $1 million from the Illinois Department of Commerce and Community Affairs. These funds were allocated to hire a support staff (one-third of the funding) and to launch a small grants program (two-thirds of the funding). Between 1987 and 1992, the amount of federal funding to the involved departments increased from $3.5 million per year to $10 million annually. Since 1992, there has been no significant growth, and the consortium has been deemphasized in the research efforts of involved departments (although it continues to offer some regional collaboration in graduate medical education). Dr. Robert deVito (chair of the board of directors of the consortium and chair of psychiatry at Loyola Medical School) and Dr. Boris Astrachan (chair of psychiatry at the University of Illinois–Chicago) both highlighted the early optimism, the failure to complete a major recruitment of two senior drug abuse researchers, and the departure of several of the chairs as critical to the loss of momentum. Ultimately, the consortium structure was neither focused enough to develop a common research enterprise nor structured enough to accept federal grants (and indirect costs). The latter probably would have been discouraged by the parent universities and medical schools, which had existing structures for research administration.

Another model of regional collaboration was developed by substance abuse researchers at Yale and the University of Connecticut (UConn). In the FY 1994 data, the department of psychiatry at the University of Connecticut was in the top quartile of NIH research support, in a medical school at the top of the bottom half. As described by Dr. Thomas Babor (interim chair), "a major part of the department's research has been focused on the addictions" (T. F. Babor, personal communication, June 1996). In 1978 the department received a center grant from NIAAA that helped to establish it, at the time, as the only major research group in the country integrating basic and clinical research on the etiology and treatment of alcoholism. Currently the Alcohol Research Center (ARC) is supported by a center grant from NIAAA (21% of the ARC budget), investigator-initiated grants (43% of the budget), and two cooperative agreements with NIAAA (23% of the budget). The latter grants have brought the ARC into active collaboration with researchers in human genetics and with health services researchers at other universities across the United States.

Commencing in 1986, the ARC at UConn and the addiction research programs at the Connecticut Mental Health Center and the West Haven VA Medical Center at Yale established a "center without walls" consisting of more than 50 senior addiction scientists between the two universities (located 35 miles apart). "Interlocking collaborative agreements have been developed by means of mutual advisory committees and interinstitutional research grants" (T. F. Babor, personal communication, June 1996). A NIDA-funded center grant to Yale funds a component at UConn, while the NIAAA-funded center at UConn funds some research at Yale.

"Clinical facilities, scientific investigators and research laboratories can be matched to the needs of a given project. . . . On the national level, with the dramatic improvements in communications technologies, and the growing complexity of research designs, there is a movement toward 'big science' that brings collaborating groups together across institutional lines" (T. F. Babor, personal communication, June 1996). By linking a group of able investigators at a university with a relatively spare infrastructure for psychiatric research to investigators at other universities with access to important technology, the department of psychiatry at UConn has been able to maintain its edge in alcoholism and addiction research and its place in the top quartile of research departments of psychiatry. In the late 1980s and early 1990s the department was able to parlay the reputation of the ARC to secure some state funds to retain promising investigators with the award of tenure.

The decade-long collaboration among investigators at Yale and UConn has survived because it fosters a collaborative spirit among junior and senior investigators in both research centers. Grant funds flowed under subcontracts in both directions. The model was not mandated from top-down but has continued to grow and change with the addition of faculty in both places. More particularly, it continues to thrive despite the fact that the original leaders of the research activity in the addictions at Yale and UConn are no longer on the scene. Neither of the research administrative offices at the universities have discouraged the collaboration, in spite of the greater complexity involved in the administration of grants with subcontracts.

The University of Connecticut example also serves to highlight the importance of developing special niche areas of research expertise as a vehicle for success in relatively high-achieving departments. In its 1989 survey of the research activities of full-time psychiatry faculty (Pincus et al. 1993), the APA's office of research found that more than 45% of physician researchers were primarily interested in schizophrenia, affective disorders, or anxiety disorders. Only 3.2% identified themselves as drug abuse researchers, 4.1% as alcoholism researchers, 8.2% as researchers interested in geriatric psychiatric disorders, and 6.9% as researchers of child and adolescent psychiatry as their primary area of interest. NIMH funds all of these research areas, but other NIH institutes also fund drug abuse, alcoholism, aging, and child development research. Health services research has been mandated to be part of the research portfolios of the three former ADAMHA institutes. Only 2.3% of physician researchers in the survey identified themselves as health services researchers.

Among the high-achieving psychiatry departments, Connecticut, SUNY–Brooklyn, Medical University of South Carolina, Wayne State, and the University of Oklahoma have all developed significant research programs in alcoholism or addictions. The University of Miami has a major program in AIDS research funded by NIMH, which also funds important AIDS research programs in psychiatry departments at Columbia and the University of California–San Francisco. The University of Arkansas has developed a major program in health services research, along with a clinical research program at its affiliated Veterans Administration (VA) medical center. George Washington University has a premier program of research on family process that has been collaboratively linked to distinguished behavioral genetics researchers at other universities in the United States and abroad. Departments lacking critical technology (as in behavioral genetics at George Washington or at the University of Connecticut) established linkages with researchers at other universities. Many high-achieving departments have been successful because they have developed strong niches outside of the traditional areas of research on schizophrenia, affective disorders, and anxiety disorders. Indeed, a number of NIH institutes (e.g., National Cancer Institute [NCI], National Heart, Lung, and Blood Institute [NHLBI], National Institute of Child Health and Development [NICHD], and National Institute on Aging [NIA]) fund programs in behavioral medicine or human development tied to research programs in psychiatry departments.

Three other general issues stand out in considering the research success of psychiatry departments: 1) the research center grant mechanism, 2) the willingness of some universities to reward productive research programs with financial credits for grant-related savings on faculty salary support or indirect cost recovery, and 3) the collaborative grant mechanisms of NIH and the Department of Veterans Affairs. Research centers supported by NIMH, NIDA, and NIAAA have provided a framework for training young investigators, fostering collaboration of basic and clinical scientists within (and among) AHCs, fostering support for shared resources and scientific infrastructure in the psychiatry department and the AHC, and providing a framework for the conduct of essential longitudinal studies related to risk factors and the course of illness. *The center grant mechanism is critical to the future of psychiatric research.*

A number of research-intensive departments have benefited from center grants and the ability to "multiply" grant-related support through institutional awards based on grant-related income. The latter has enabled departments to stabilize salary support for young investigators, to support the collection of pilot data for new grant submissions, and to otherwise support the research infrastructure for psychiatry. Finally, the collaborative grant mechanism has been responsible for large-scale clinical trials and pedigree studies that have helped to advance psychopharmacology, psychotherapy research, and major genetics studies. It has been a critical foundation for clinical research and clinical trials in psychiatry.

One of the more remarkable success stories in developing a research enterprise comes from Dallas, Texas. As described by Dr. Kern Wildenthal (Association of Academic Health Centers, unpublished observations, 1996, p. 2), "the most successful strategy in generating funds for supporting clinical and basic research at UT Southwestern has 'recently' been to seek gifts from the community." Between 1943 and 1985, the endowment of the University of Texas–Southwestern (UT Southwestern) had grown to only $35 million. By 1995, as a result of an intensive development effort, the endowment reached $265 million. In 1985, the development office had "one secretary who wrote and typed letters of appreciation for any gifts that arrived." By 1995 the development budget had grown to $600,000, less than 2% of philanthropic income. The school has focused its efforts with "local foundations, businesses, and individuals whose primary motives for giving . . . [include] general altruism, the desire to conquer disease and civic pride." As the only medical school in Dallas, the institution has devoted "considerable attention to building its image and level of awareness in the community." The extraordinary local philanthropic support for programs in the department of psychiatry at UT Southwestern must be seen in the context of the school's efforts, as well as the special skills and efforts of the

department chair, Dr. Kenneth Altshuler. Both the department of psychiatry and the school of medicine are ranked in their respective top
quartiles of research support from NIH.

When Dr. Altshuler became chair in 1977, the department had few
psychiatrists, few psychologists, and a residency training program on
probation. "It was clear to me that to build a department of any stature,
I would need to raise research funds . . . to attract . . . able investigators. It was also clear that I had to turn to the private sector, since the
public sector was shrinking . . . and . . . Texas (was) 48th out of 50
states in per capita spending" for the mentally ill (in the public sector).
"Accordingly, I set out to meet as many people as I could and to do as
many favors as I possibly could, primarily in helping people to find the
. . . services they would need. . . . I was frequently called by total
strangers, and I tried to meet people who had an impact in the City
(and) offered to be at their service should such unfortunate needs ever
arise. . . . I had the great good fortune to meet early a couple of won-
derful individuals": the president of a bank who also headed two foundations and a leading philanthropist and volunteer. "Meeting with each
of these individuals . . . , each of whom had a brush with illness in their
family, led to having each embrace my cause," a research focus for the
department of psychiatry in the city's only medical school (K. Z. Altshuler, personal communication, May 1996).

In all, over the past 19 years, Dr. Altshuler has raised funds for nine
endowed chairs, two distinguished professorships, one professorship, a
lectureship, plus other assorted research funds of $18 million. It is a
remarkable story. Dr. Altshuler notes that he was unable to generate
the same sort of philanthropic interest in the Dallas Psychoanalytic Institute that he was able to develop for the biological research programs
in the department of psychiatry. In the end, he was also able to secure
some public-sector funding for research to improve outcomes for the
chronically mentally ill. The latter program is a public sector–academic
partnership.

Finally, no review of the recent research successes of academic psychiatry would be complete without considering the unique position of
the psychiatry department at the University of Pittsburgh. Under the
leadership of Dr. Thomas Detre, who became chair in the early 1970s,
and Dr. David Kupfer, who assumed the chair in the early 1980s follow-

ing his role as associate chair for research, the department's research programs have blossomed across the full span of research on mental and addictive disorders. As described earlier, at $39 million per year in NIH support, the department's grant support is the most of any research-intensive psychiatry department in the United States.

In a recent communication (October 1996), Dr. Kupfer notes that for more than two decades "one of the major goals of (the) department . . . has . . . been to create new knowledge . . . and to train young investigators to conduct basic and clinical research." These goals can be achieved only if the department funds the type of infrastructure that can provide "necessary resources and resource allocations." The infrastructure "must . . . facilitate the initiation of grants . . . and overall mentoring [including] continuous grant reviewing internal to the department. . . . A 'well functioning' research committee and specialized clusters with sufficient expertise (e.g., geriatrics, child psychiatry) as well as an internal grants office, are essential. . . . Both basic and clinical research programs require that the administration assure adequate space, personnel, and administrative facilitation of the implementation of grants. . . . In the clinical arena, one needs to provide connections to clinical delivery systems such that the referral of patients and subjects are . . . well integrated into [the overall system]. Resource development also needs to provide liaisons with those centralized facilities of the medical center such as functional neuroimaging and animal laboratories, but it also must provide certain centralized facilities within [the] department." The environment should be "competitive . . . [with] incentives to collaborate and disincentives to be a 'Lone Ranger.' " "Although the R-01 is the heart of what most of us do, one needs to maintain the position that in certain areas it is important to develop centers of excellence [that] . . . can provide the environment in which new ideas and new investigators can emerge from post-doctoral research training programs." The department has benefited from "an adequate mixture of physicians and non-physicians." Dr. Kupfer concludes with the statement that "sustained nurturance from departmental leadership is crucial if such an endeavor is to succeed over several decades."

The quote offered by David Kupfer is a good statement of the research culture at Pittsburgh, *which has benefited substantially from a well-structured relationship with the public sector and the ability to access indirect cost funding from grants to strengthen the research infrastructure in psychiatry.* Both of these arrangements were wisely negotiated with the relevant parties by Dr. Detre when he assumed the chair in the 1970s. The department has been able to develop strong research programs in mainstream areas of psychiatry (mood disorders and schizophrenia), as well as in critical niche areas such as aging, psychiatric epidemiology, services research, child psychiatry, and drug and alcohol addiction. It is the only psychiatry department with separately funded research centers from NIDA and NIAAA. In short, as one might predict, the most successful research department in American psychiatry has all of the elements of success in one place. It resides in a medical school in the top quartile of research support, it derives a moderate amount of funding from the public sector, it is able to access indirect-cost grant support for its research infrastructure, and it has a broadly based research portfolio that draws on the resources of a number of NIH institutes.

Summary

In many respects, the extraordinary growth of psychiatric research over the past 15 years is one of the great success stories in American medicine and in the history of American psychiatry. Its success is owed to a number of factors that have served to make research a major concern to the leadership in the field, to key citizen-advocacy organizations, and to the federal government. Some departments are part of schools with strong research traditions and an infrastructure that may include a small grants program, shared research resources, a clinical research center, functional brain imaging, human genetics, behavioral neurobiology, and other disciplines and resources relevant to modern psychiatric research. The availability of center grants from NIH and of funding by foundations with a commitment to psychiatric research has also contributed to the success of the stronger research departments of psychiatry. The ability of some departments to access funding from grant-related indirect cost support to strengthen their research infrastructures has been a critical asset, but the vitality of the research enterprise for a number of departments of psychiatry rests on a continuing linkage of public-sector support to the research activities of the academic department.

In addition, as new and improved technologies become available for brain science, the field will need to be certain that a new generation of investigators is capable of applying these tools in realistic ways to research on psychiatric disorders. These investigators will need to be clinically and scientifically sophisticated. The future depends on the awareness and support of the research infrastructure by the leaders of academic medical centers and by the federal government. It calls for creative strategies to facilitate collaboration between basic biological, behavioral, and social scientists and clinical investigators within and among universities.

References

Association of Academic Health Centers: The End of an Era of Cross Subsidization of Research: A Case Study of the University of Texas Southwestern Medical Center at Dallas. Washington, DC, Association of Academic Health Centers, 1996

Burnett DA: Evolving market will change clinical research. Health Affairs 15(suppl 3):90–92, 1996

Institute of Medicine: Alcoholism, Alcohol Abuse and Related Problems: Opportunities for Research. Washington, DC, National Academy Press, 1980

Institute of Medicine, National Academy of Sciences: Research on Mental Illness and Addictive Disorders: Progress and Prospects. Washington, DC, National Academy Press, 1984

Institute of Medicine, National Academy of Sciences: Personnel and Training Needs for Biomedical and Behavioral Research. Washington, DC, National Academy Press, 1985

Institute of Medicine: Causes and Consequences of Alcohol Problems: An Agenda for Research. Washington, DC, National Academy Press, 1987

Institute of Medicine: Research on Children and Adolescents with Mental, Behavioral and Developmental Disorders. Washington, DC, National Academy Press, 1989a

Institute of Medicine: Report of a Study: Prevention and Treatment of Alcohol Problems: Research Opportunities. Washington, DC, National Academy Press, 1989b

Institute of Medicine: Pathways of Addiction: Opportunities in Drug Abuse Research. Washington, DC, National Academy Press, 1996

Kessler RC, McGonagle KA, Zhao S, et al: Lifetime and 12-month prevalence of DSM-III R psychiatric disorders in the United States: results from the National Comorbidity Survey. Arch Gen Psychiatry 51:8–19, 1994

Levey GS, Sherman CR, Gentile NO, et al: Postdoctoral research training of full-time faculty in academic departments of medicine. Ann Intern Med 109:414–418, 1988

Mechanic R, Dobson A: Managed care and clinical research. Health Affairs 15:72–89, 1996

Pincus HA, Fine T: The anatomy of research funding of mental illness and addictive disorders. Arch Gen Psychiatry 49:573–579, 1992

Pincus HA, Dial TH, Haviland MG: Research activities of full-time faculty in academic departments of psychiatry. Arch Gen Psychiatry 50:657–664, 1993

Regier DA, Boyd JH, Burke JD Jr, et al: One-month prevalence of mental disorders in the United States. Arch Gen Psychiatry 45:977–986, 1988

CHAPTER 5

Psychiatry and the New Emphasis on Primary Care

Roger E. Meyer, M.D., and Christopher J. McLaughlin

Starting in the 1950s, the balance of influence within American medicine shifted from general practice to medical and surgical subspecialties. Other physicians and patients presumed that specialists were more knowledgeable and skillful than generalists, and the educational programs within academic health centers reinforced the view that if you were truly sick, you should be cared for by a specialist with access to the latest technology and scientific information. During this period, primary care disciplines struggled for legitimacy within the hierarchy of values of the academic health center.[1] With regard to mental disorders, it was felt that a significant percentage of patients being cared for by general practitioners were emotionally ill, and probably better served by psychiatrists. The long workdays of the generalists, combined with the prevalence of psychiatric problems among their patients, encouraged a number of general practitioners to be retrained as psychiatrists during the 1950s through early 1970s.

It is interesting, 30 to 40 years later, to read a new literature focusing on the high prevalence of psychiatric disorders and subthreshold symp-

---

[1] According to Block et al. (1996), this is still a problem.

tom clusters in primary care practices (see later section) and describing the problem of burnout among the practitioners (deGruy 1996). Certainly, the problem of the most effective way to treat mental disorders in primary care practices is still present. Moreover, this issue will only grow more urgent as managed health care emphasizes the generalist as the cornerstone of the health care system. If 40 years of history are to be instructive, it is clear that the integration of mental and general health care for real patients will require a greater degree of collaboration than ever before among psychiatrists, other mental health professionals, primary care physicians, and other primary care clinicians.

While the educational programs in psychiatry and in primary care disciplines have traditionally emphasized a humanistic message of caring, there have been few examples of authentic interdepartmental collaboration in the education of medical students, residents, and physicians in practice. Rather than engage faculty from the psychiatry department, departments of family medicine have been more likely to hire their own behavioral scientists to teach residents about the diagnosis and management of mental disorders and subthreshold emotional symptoms. Conversely, psychiatry departments have emphasized bedside teaching around complex medical and psychiatric comorbidity as the focal point of their consultation services. The latter has been the usual point of interface between psychiatry and other departments in the academic health center (AHC), and it communicated a bias consistent with the specialist orientation of the medical center. There was a failure to appreciate the value system of primary care clinicians. These values are exemplified in the following definition of primary care adopted by the Institute of Medicine (IOM) Committee on the Future of Primary Care: "Primary care is the provision of *integrated, accessible health care services* by *clinicians* who are *accountable* for addressing a large *majority of personal health care needs,* developing a *sustained partnership with patients,* and practicing in the *context of family and community* [italics mine]" (Donaldson et al. 1994, p. 1).

For psychiatry to interface more effectively with the clinical and educational mission of academic primary care disciplines, and for psychiatric clinicians to interface more effectively with their primary care colleagues, the field will need to come to terms with the new centrality of primary care in the transformation of the health care system. As summarized by the IOM Committee on the Future of Primary Care, "primary care can address a large majority of the health problems present in the population" (Donaldson et al. 1994, p. 36). The report argues that primary care physicians can serve the needs of health promotion, disease prevention, and care of the chronically ill, through integrated health care delivery systems and long-standing personal relationships with patients to promote a high quality of care, high degree of patient satisfaction, and substantial cost efficiencies.

For psychiatrists, who have also emphasized high-quality doctor-patient relationships as the foundation stone of effective psychotherapeutic care, the perceived transfer of long-term ambulatory treatment to primary care physicians represents a substantial paradigm shift. However, as described later in this chapter, if primary care physicians are to work more effectively on behalf of their patients with mental disorders, they will need to gain new skills and knowledge and develop practice patterns that can better integrate health and mental health care. Both psychiatrists and primary care physicians will be challenged to incorporate new research findings into practice, in the context of managed care systems that are concerned about maximum throughput and costs of care.

Mental Disorders and Emotional Symptoms in Primary Care Practice

It is generally acknowledged that a substantial percentage of patients seen in primary care settings have diagnosable mental disorders. More than 15 years ago, the National Institute of Mental Health (NIMH) Epidemiological Catchment Area Study reported that a greater percentage of adult patients with mental disorders are treated solely in a general health care setting (45.1%) versus a specialized mental health treatment setting (38.4%) (Regier et al. 1978). More recently, using a diagnostic instrument developed for primary care practice, Spitzer and colleagues (1995) and Johnson et al. (1995) found that one or more disorders were diagnosed in 39% of 1,000 patients seen in four primary care sites. One-third of these patients had only a subthreshold diagnosis, such as minor depression or anxiety disorder (not otherwise specified).

While these diagnoses did not meet formal DSM-III-R (American Psychiatric Association 1987) diagnostic criteria, they were associated with considerable impairment. The most prevalent disorders identified in this cohort were mood disorder (26%), anxiety disorder (18%), somatoform disorder (14%), alcohol use disorder (5%), and eating disorder (3%). Consistent with other studies (Hays et al. 1995), depressive disorders in the primary care setting were associated with substantial functional impairment.[2] In the study reported by Spitzer et al. (1995), significant impairment was also found among patients with anxiety, somatoform, and eating disorders.

Utilizing another diagnostic system designed to screen for psychiatric disorders and subthreshold psychiatric symptoms in primary care settings, Olfson et al. (1996) reported that 30.1% of 1,001 patients seen in a primary care practice at Kaiser Permanente in Oakland, California, met criteria for subthreshold symptoms, and 38.9% of these patients also met criteria for an Axis I mental disorder. Olfson et al. found a similar range of psychiatric disorders and subthreshold conditions as in the study by Spitzer and colleagues (1996) but found substantial impairment associated only with depressive and panic symptoms. Differences in level of impairment found in the two studies could be a function of different patient samples, different psychiatric screening instruments, different criteria for subthreshold disorders, or the use of different instruments to assess level of function or impairment. The relevant conclusion across a growing list of epidemiologic studies in primary care settings is that despite important methodological differences, there is a significant prevalence of psychiatric disorders and subthreshold conditions that can impact on quality of life measures and the costs of medical care (Henk et al. 1996).[3]

Patients with mental disorders usually present to a primary care clinician with a physical complaint (Bridges and Goldberg 1985; Kroenke et al. 1994). As a consequence, these patients tend to utilize more

---

[2] The level of impairment associated with depression in the latter study generally exceeded that found with other common medical conditions.

[3] Indeed, where there is comorbidity of psychiatric conditions and some medical disorders (hypertension and diabetes), there is more functional impairment associated with the medical disorders than in patients with the medical disorder alone (Sherbourne et al. 1996).

medical resources than other patients in the primary care practice (McFarland et al. 1985; Shapiro et al. 1984). Patients with somatization disorder (Barsky and Borus 1995) and panic disorder (Katon 1996) are especially likely to use more medical resources. Smith (1994) has reported that patients with somatization disorder utilize nine times the resources of the typical primary care patient. Among patients with negative findings on coronary angiograms or radiologic or endoscopic evaluation of the bowel, the prevalence of panic disorder may be 30 to 40 times that observed in the community (Katon 1996). There is also an extremely high prevalence of panic disorder among patients with unexplained neurological symptoms (Katon 1996).

In a system at financial risk from the overuse of diagnostic and other services, or from the failure to diagnose serious treatable illnesses, the ability to differentiate somatizing patients without significant nonpsychiatric medical pathology from such patients with significant pathology should be a high priority. Under capitation, providers have incentives to decrease utilization and as a result somatizers may urgently exaggerate their symptomatology to a succession of physicians (Barsky and Borus 1995). In prepaid plans, somatizers have little incentive to not seek medical attention. The situation is complicated because between one-third and two-thirds of primary care patients with a psychiatric diagnosis also have significant nonpsychiatric medical conditions (Cartwright 1967; Garfield et al. 1976; Hilkevitch 1965; Lipowski 1988).

Howard et al. (1996) have reported that many persons with mental illness begin the process of treatment through nonpsychiatric physicians, who provide almost half of all mental health services. While these authors reported that 23% of the office hours of primary care physicians are spent in mental health service delivery, Rosenblatt (1995) reported that less than 3% of the average caseload of the primary care clinicians is devoted to mental health care. These seemingly discrepant findings are consistent with the view that patients with mental disorders or significant subthreshold symptomatology tend to utilize proportionately more of a general physician's time than other patients in the caseload. Thus, while deGruy (1996, p. 102) has emphasized that "mental health care is only a part of primary care practice," interventions that might improve the cost-effectiveness of this component of primary care practice could make a substantial difference in the lives of primary care physicians and their patients (Smith et al. 1986, 1995). Within the academic health center anxious to develop a cost-efficient network of primary care clinicians, efforts to integrate psychiatric and general health care within primary care practices could improve the cost-effectiveness of primary care services. Capitation rates (or charges) for primary care services would need to calculate the contribution of each component of the health care team, and the management of the practice would need to assure equitable reimbursement across collaborating departments and faculty.

Nonrecognition and Undertreatment of Psychiatric Disorders and Subthreshold Symptomatology in Primary Care Practice

Primary care physicians are usually oriented to respond to a chief complaint. Because the average primary care visit lasts 13 minutes (Bryant and Shimizu 1988), there is often little time for an interview that might yield more specific diagnostic information or details on the environmental context or meaning of the patient's symptoms. DeGruy (1996) has listed a number of factors that discourage recognition of mental disorders in primary care settings. These factors include patient resistance to accepting a diagnosis of mental disorder, patient presentation with significant somatization, the rapid pace of primary care practice, the focus on the chief complaint rather than psychosocial material within the history-taking interview, diagnostic systems that do not fit the clinical phenomenology, problems with reimbursement, and lack of knowledge and skills on the part of the primary physician.

Most of the recent efforts to enhance the quality of mental health services delivery in primary care settings have focused on 1) new iterations of criteria of psychiatric disorders around algorithms oriented to primary care practice; 2) improved screening instruments geared to the manifestations of psychiatric disorders or subthreshold conditions in this milieu; 3) enhanced case-oriented psychiatric or mental health consultation in the general health care environment; 4) the teaching of practice guidelines skills to the generalist; and 5) the incorporation of cognitive, educational, and behavioral treatments by nonphysician mental or be-havioral health service providers into the primary care practice.

At this writing, there appears to be good consensus that between one-half and two-thirds of patients meeting criteria for mental disorders go unrecognized in primary care practices (Higgins 1994). Even where physician recognition of mood and anxiety disorders has been enhanced through the use of screening instruments, recognition was not sufficient to assure the treatment of these disorders in accordance with clinical guidelines (Tiemens et al. 1996). Sturm and Wells (1995) have dem-onstrated that the treatment of depression is more effective when pro-vided by psychiatrists in a mental health setting than when given by primary care physicians in a general health care practice, but they also suggest that more cost-effective care might result from shifting some patients from psychiatrists to general physicians, with attention to quality-improvement measures.

To some extent the problems in the primary care practices involved inadequate dosage and duration of antidepressant treatment (Sturm and Wells 1995), but patient compliance with treatment recommendations could also be an issue. Katon et al. (1995, 1996) were able to demon-strate enhanced compliance by depressed patients in primary care set-tings when practice guidelines were reinforced by the ready availability of mental health consultation in those settings.[4] These conclusions are similar to recommendations made in the review by deGruy (1996). DeGruy proposed a relevant alignment of mental health consultation and direct services to improve the diagnosis and treatment of mental disorders in primary care practice. This approach would require greater collaboration and understanding of the realities of the general practice environment by psychiatrists and of standards of best practice for mental disorders by primary care clinicians. Ultimately, the enhancement of screening efficacy for mental disorders in primary care practice can only be helpful if it is linked to effective treatment that is not usually available in most of these settings. The costs of the mental or behavioral health consultation, intervention, and oversight probably cannot be covered by

---

[4] Because the spontaneous recovery rate of patients with minor depression was high, the multifaceted intervention advocated by these investigators was found to be more effective with more seriously depressed patients.

discounted fee-for-service billing by these clinicians but might be incorporated in bundled charges for primary health care services.

A Diagnostic System for Mental Disorders in Primary Care Settings

It is generally acknowledged that primary care physicians need screening and assessment tools that are user-friendly if they are to recognize the principal mental disorders and symptoms that present in their practices. The DSM-IV–PC (American Psychiatric Association 1995b) was developed by representatives of the principal primary care organizations and the American Psychiatric Association to translate current psychiatric diagnostic nomenclature into a manual for primary care clinicians. The manual is divided into four sections. Section 1 describes disorders and conditions most frequently encountered in primary care, including depressed mood, anxiety, unexplained general medical symptoms, cognitive disturbance, problematic substance use, sleep disturbance, sexual dysfunction, weight change or abnormal eating, and psychotic symptoms. This section of the manual (algorithms of mental disorders) is organized by presenting symptoms. Each algorithm includes a series of steps to guide the clinician to consider diagnostic options. An introductory text accompanies each algorithm and focuses on epidemiology, the presentation of symptoms in primary care, differential diagnosis in common associated conditions, and the organization of the algorithm.

The second section describes the types of psychosocial problems encountered in primary care practice, including relational or family problems, problems related to abuse or neglect, and difficulties in personal or social roles. This section also includes physiological and behavioral factors that may affect health care. The third section describes disorders that are rarely first identified in primary care, including manic symptoms, impulse control problems, deviant sexual arousal, dissociative symptoms, abnormal movements or vocalizations, and dysfunctional personality traits. The final section of the manual deals with mental disorders usually first diagnosed in childhood or adolescence. As described by Pincus et al. (1995), the manual was designed to be relevant to primary care practice and compatible with DSM-IV (American Psychiatric Association 1995a), but it is probably most useful as a framework for collaboration between primary care physicians and consultation psychiatrists.

Screening Instruments

A number of authors have suggested the usefulness of brief self-report screening instruments for mental disorders in general health care settings (Higgins 1994; Spitzer et al. 1995). In their report on quality of life measures in primary care patients with mental disorders, Spitzer and co-workers (1995) recommended that computer-scored forms could be incorporated into routine practice. As an indirect measure of psychiatric symptomatology, they specifically endorsed the patient self-administered brief screening instruments that had been developed for the Medical Outcomes Study of health-related quality of life (Stewart et al. 1989; Wells et al. 1989). The PRIME-MD is another brief questionnaire designed to improve the detection of common mental disorders in primary care practice (Spitzer et al. 1994). It includes 25 questions dealing with mood, anxiety, alcohol, eating, and somatoform disorders. Although the overall usefulness and extent of utilization of the instrument in primary care practices is somewhat controversial (Maurer 1996), free copies of the instrument are being made available by Pfizer Pharmaceuticals. At this juncture, screening for mental disorders in primary care settings is still at a relatively early stage of development. A new generation of screening instruments will need to be tested for sensitivity, specificity, reliability, and validity, as well as cost-effectiveness, in this milieu.[5]

There is actually better data on screening for alcohol problems in primary care practice than for other mental disorders. The CAGE questions were designed to identify alcoholic patients in medical settings by focusing on the respondent's lifetime drinking history (Ewing 1984;

---

[5] While there is experience with self-report and clinician-completed rating scales for depression in primary care practice, they have a high false-positive rate relative to the identification of major depressive disorder. Clinicians are then encouraged to conduct a psychiatric assessment sufficient to establish the presence or absence of a DSM-IV disorder.

Mayfield et al. 1974). Because the four questions can be asked in about 1 minute, the instrument is very user-friendly for primary care physicians, but the questions may not be sensitive enough to detect *problem drinking* (as in older patients) (Adams et al. 1996). The MAST, an instrument consisting of 25 questions, was also developed to identify alcoholics in general health care settings (Selzer 1971). It has been adapted to a briefer format (10 or 13 questions) and for patient self-administration (Pokorny et al. 1972; Selzer et al. 1975; Swenson and Morese 1975). Both the CAGE and the MAST have demonstrated their validity in the identification of alcoholism in inpatient and outpatient medical settings over the past 20 years.

The AUDIT was developed for a World Health Organization (WHO) study of early identification of, and brief interventions to counter, alcohol problems in primary care settings (Babor and Grant 1989). The AUDIT is a 10-question instrument. In the WHO study, its overall sensitivity was 92%, and its specificity was 93%. By focusing on the screening of alcohol problems rather than alcohol dependence and providing primary care physicians with brief intervention tools compatible with the pace of primary care practice—and the generic needs of patients to increase their awareness of a hazardous lifestyle and to learn alternative coping skills—the WHO study was able to demonstrate some effectiveness in altering hazardous or harmful drinking patterns in primary care patients. If it had focused on the identification of alcohol dependence, it would have identified cases that required referral to a specialized treatment service, since there is no evidence that brief interventions are useful in alcohol-dependent individuals. The study should also be instructive to those who wish to simply increase the screening efficacy for all mental disorders in primary care settings. Screening is useful if it enables the clinician to practice more efficiently and appropriately and if it helps to assure that the patient receives the most cost-effective treatment.

Finally, screening for alcohol, illicit drugs, tobacco, and general health risks can be incorporated into self- or physician-administered general health screening instruments (Fleming and Barry 1991). Since physicians may be reluctant to ask patients some of these questions, especially during a planned brief visit, general health screening instruments may have great utility in routine practice. If educators in primary care and psychiatry are able to develop some collaborative training programs for medical students and residents, both fields would be well served by a greater understanding of the prospects and limitations of various screening instruments in the identification of mental symptoms, disorders, and problem behaviors in the primary care setting.

Improving the Quality of Mental Health Care in Primary Care Practice

While there is much interest in problems of identification and treatment of a number of mental disorders in primary care practice, the best outcome data relates to the identification and treatment of major depressive disorder. The Agency for Health Care Policy and Research (AHCPR) has developed a brief, two-volume edition of clinical practice guidelines developed by an expert panel consisting of primary care physicians, consultation psychiatrists, one health services researcher, and one research psychiatrist (Depression Guideline Panel 1993a,b). The first volume focuses on detection and diagnosis and the second volume on treatment. A recent report compared the outcomes of patients treated according to AHCPR guidelines with those given usual treatment by the patient's primary care physician (Schulberg et al. 1996). Despite being counseled by the study team to inform their physicians of their mood disorder, the members of the team discovered that either patients were not communicating with their physicians or they were not receiving requested help. The team then felt it necessary to intervene directly with the physicians about the patients' psychiatric diagnoses. Despite these extra efforts, patients receiving usual treatment did significantly less well than patients receiving either the AHCPR-recommended dose and duration of nortriptyline or the recommended course of interpersonal psychotherapy administered by trained psychologists or psychiatrists at the primary care site.

The authors concluded that motivated primary care physicians can be trained to prescribe antidepressant medication to achieve outcomes as good as those psychiatrists can obtain with these drugs, but it was unclear whether primary care physicians would be able to routinely adopt the practice guidelines for detection, diagnosis, and treatment recommended by AHCPR. In a companion article in the same issue of the *Archives of General Psychiatry,* another team of health service researchers found that while almost all depressed patients treated by mental health specialists in their study received at least brief counseling, less than half of the depressed patients in the general medical sector received such counseling. The situation was worse for patients in prepaid than in fee-for-service care in the primary care practice (Meredith et al. 1996).

Although it is too soon to draw definitive conclusions, it would appear that efforts to improve the quality of mental health care in primary care settings will require a major investment of resources. Optimally this approach would include patient education, the use of didactic materials and case consultations in the education of primary care physicians, and on-site, experienced mental health professionals who can provide counseling or brief therapy to patients and feedback on the patients' course to their primary care physicians (Katon et al. 1995, 1996). Optimal care of depressed patients can remain in the primary care setting, but only by making substantial changes in that setting. Other studies are needed to determine whether this type of effort would be useful in the treatment of patients with other common psychiatric and substance use disorders.

At this juncture, academic psychiatrists and primary care physicians should feel both reassured and challenged. In an optimal system, the roles and responsibilities of each discipline would be greatly enhanced— but such an undertaking will require substantial collaboration. Unfortunately, in many academic health centers, there is little evidence of the type of clinical or educational collaboration between these disciplines that would be necessary to advance the opportunity to develop high-quality mental health services in primary care settings.

Academic Psychiatry and the Education of Primary Care Physicians

There is a long history of exhortative articles urging psychiatrists to play a more active role in the education of primary care physicians. The problem with this literature, as critiqued by deGruy (1996), is that there is no agreement between psychiatrists and primary care physicians about what should be learned, who should teach it, and how the relationship between the disciplines should be structured. One place to begin the process of education is defining the proposed skills (and consequent roles) of the primary care practitioner. Table 5–1 lists the skills that 46 responding psychiatry department chairs felt that primary care physicians should have relative to the care of mental disorders in their practices. Despite the literature (cited earlier) that highlights the deficiencies of primary care practitioners in making psychiatric diagnoses and prescribing antidepressant drugs, there is surprising support among a strong majority of these department heads that primary care physicians should have the skills to make DSM-IV diagnoses, refer to a psychiatrist or other mental health professional, perform risk assessment, and prescribe anxiolytics and antidepressants. A minority also believe that primary care physicians could perform counseling, offer maintenance treatment of chronic mental illness, or prescribe medications for psychotic patients (schizophrenia or bipolar disorder) or alcoholics.

We do not have comparable survey responses from heads of primary care programs, but Table 5–2 contrasts the responses of the heads of the psychiatry departments and the principal adult primary care pro-

TABLE 5-1

Psychiatric services to be provided by primary care physicians as reported by 46 responding psychiatry department chairs

Service	Percentage responding that service could be provided by primary care physicians
Counseling	39
Diagnosis using DSM-IV	72
Maintenance of the chronically mentally ill	30
Primary care of the mentally ill	67
Referral to a psychiatrist	93
Referral to a mental health professional	89
Risk assessment	74
Treatment with antidepressants	85
Treatment with anxiolytics	85
Treatment with mood-stabilizing drugs	26
Treatment with naltrexone for alcoholism	39
Treatment with neuroleptics	33

TABLE 5-2

Psychiatry services to be provided by primary care physicians reported
by primary care and psychiatry department chairs at five case study
institutions*

Service	Number of primary care chairs responding	Number of psychiatry chairs responding
Counseling	5	3
Diagnosis using DSM-IV	4	3
Maintenance of the chronically mentally ill	5	1
Primary care of the mentally ill	5	3
Referral to a psychiatrist	5	5
Referral to a mental health professional	5	4
Risk assessment	5	5
Treatment with antidepressants	5	3
Treatment with anxiolytics	5	4
Treatment with mood-stabilizing drugs	2	2
Treatment with naltrexone for alcoholism	4	1
Treatment with neuroleptics	1	2

*Stanford, Maryland, Colorado, Louisville, and Dartmouth

grams at the five case study academic health centers. In general, virtually
all of the primary care program directors endorsed all of the skills
categories except the use of mood-stabilizing drugs or antipsychotic
medication.

The data suggest that some academic leaders in primary care believe
that they can provide all mental health services, except acute treatment
of the seriously mentally ill. The individual case studies actually highlight
subtle differences in tone. Despite strong interest from the psychiatry
chair in collaborative education, the head of family practice at Colorado
was most emphatic about the skills of his faculty and their ability to
teach their own residents about mental disorders without input from
psychiatry. In contrast, the heads of family practice at Maryland and of
internal medicine at Dartmouth welcomed the presence of psychiatry
faculty in the practice milieu. The head of general internal medicine at
Stanford wanted more input from psychiatry than was being provided
by a senior resident.

Table 5–3 lists the educational methods used by the 46 responding psychiatry departments with regard to the primary care residency program. Lectures and seminars were provided by 32 of the departments. As in the survey conducted more than a decade ago by Pincus and colleagues (1983), case consultations are a very common mode of teaching. While 22 departments report that primary care residents rotate on psychiatry, it is not clear whether it is a required, selective, or elective rotation. In an earlier survey, Strain et al. (1984) noted six models of training for mental health skills in primary care residencies.[6] They urged departments of psychiatry to develop educational programs based on the needs of primary care patients and the culture of the primary care practice. The latter is often less concerned about the nuances of specific diagnostic categories and more concerned about generic concepts like *psychosis* or *depression* (Strain et al. 1986). DeGruy (1996) recently took this point one step further by pointing out that psychiatry's emphasis in its teaching programs on reliable diagnostic criteria and developments in neurobiology and psychopharmacology had created a vacuum for primary care clinicians. Primary care clinicians thus lack a theoretical

TABLE 5-3

Primary care training methods used by 46 responding departments of psychiatry

Method	Number of departments
Case consultation	27
Psychiatry rotation by primary care residents	22
Balint group	4
Lectures and seminars	32

[6] The six models they identified were 1) the consultation model, based on the case method; 2) the liaison model, incorporating the psychiatrist teacher as part of the medical team; 3) the bridge model, in which a psychiatrist actually serves as a member of the primary care treatment team; 4) the hybrid model, in which psychosocial teaching is provided by a psychiatrist, a behavioral scientist, and members of the primary care faculty; 5) the autonomous model, in which a psychiatrist is hired by the primary care group; and 6) the postgraduate specialty model, in which the primary care physician is trained in a psychiatric setting for 1 to 2 years.

"framework for understanding the human predicament and giving meaning to symptoms" (deGruy 1996).

As the role of psychiatry in academic health centers has become focused on difficult diagnostic decisions about seriously disturbed patients and medication consultations, "there is no coherent medical psychology that is taught in every medical school. . . . This leaves the primary care clinician without support when trying to understand and deal with the 'ordinary' mental distress, disorders, and illnesses encountered in the daily practice of primary care" (deGruy 1996). If deGruy is correct, then liaison activities and Balint groups may be more salient to primary care education about mental disorders and emotional symptoms than spot consultations and lectures by psychiatry faculty. In fact, as described by Katon et al. (1995, 1996), the optimal educational experience necessary to change physician practice in these settings would be quite broad based and presumably expensive. Unlike 20 years ago, when psychiatric training received federal support through NIMH, and primary care programs received similar support through the Health Resources Administration, there is no single source of support that could help alleviate the burden. At the core is a quality of care concern that will need to be addressed by academic health centers, primary care and psychiatry departments, and the leaders of the managed care industry.

Primary Care Services to the Chronically and Seriously Mentally III

Paralleling the difficulty of unrecognized psychiatric illness in primary care settings has been the problem of unrecognized nonpsychiatric medical disorders in psychiatric patients. It is a quality of care issue of at least equal import. At least three systematic studies (Hall et al. 1981; Koran et al. 1989; Sox et al. 1989) have demonstrated relatively high rates of medical disorders in psychiatric patients, and two of these studies demonstrated nonrecognition rates of approximately 50% (Hall et al. 1981; Sox et al. 1989).

The problems may be worse in relatively isolated psychiatric hospitals (public and private). Recently Dr. James Shore (1996), the psychiatry head at Colorado, proposed the creation of a new primary care elective curriculum within psychiatric residency programs to train a new generation of public-sector psychiatrists to be able to recognize and treat the most common medical disorders seen in a typical primary care practice. Although Shore's proposal emphasized the problems of undiagnosed and untreated medical disorders in the seriously and chronically mentally ill patients in the public sector, it is also possible that some behavioral health carveouts may exacerbate the problem for private- and public-sector patients with mental or addictive disorders. This difficulty is especially apparent if the carveout directs patients routinely to nonphysicians for their behavioral health care and if these nonphysicians are not well integrated into the general health care system.

Shore's proposal would appear to require a degree of collaboration between academic psychiatry and primary care departments at a time when the latter are not faced with a decline in qualified residency applicants. On the other hand, the development of *joint* training programs for residents interested in psychiatry and primary care might be attractive to some primary care departments and residency applicants excited about the prospects of integrated and sensitively delivered patient care. Primary care graduates of these programs would be better able to offer mental or behavioral health services in their practices, while the public-sector psychiatrists taking advantage of this elective track would be better able to offer primary care services to their patients. Unfortunately, while the proposal is timely and of great interest, it would not begin to address the present problems of undiagnosed or untreated medical disorders in chronically mentally ill patients (or in patients whose behavioral health care has been carved out without prior evaluation by a primary care physician). The issues are similar to those cited in earlier sections of this chapter: the challenge of quality improvement of behavioral and general health services through the implementation of changes in practice patterns and better integration of services.

The Challenges in Changing Physician Practice Patterns

In a Sounding Board essay in the *New England Journal of Medicine,* Greco and Eisenberg (1993) pondered the efficacy of different interventions in changing physician practice patterns. They contrasted the speed with which minimally invasive surgery has changed the nature of surgical practice with frustrated efforts to change physician behavior after the presentation of data from controlled clinical trials. They reviewed the efficacy of six general methods of changing physician practice: education, feedback, administrative rules, financial incentives, financial penalties, and efforts to engage physicians in the change process. They noted the failure of clinical practice guidelines and of traditional continuing medical education programs to change physician practices. As an alternative, efforts to disseminate guidelines to "opinion leaders" (including leading academics) was felt to be effective but quite labor intensive and expensive. "Moreover, it is unclear whether these techniques can succeed outside the research setting" (Greco and Eisenberg 1993, p. 1272).

Feedback regarding an individual physician's practice patterns relative to an external standard has been more effective than practice guidelines, but "the physicians must recognize that their practices need improvement," and they must have the ability to act with new skills and knowledge (Greco and Eisenberg 1993, p. 1272). Prospective reminders work better than retrospective feedback. Administrative interventions through regulatory mechanisms or utilization review can work under some circumstances, particularly if they are reinforced by financial incentives or penalties. However, such interventions can produce undesirable consequences if they increase the "hassle" factor. Optimally, according to Greco and Eisenberg, physicians should be involved in setting the standards for change as in continuous quality improvement efforts that strive to improve quality and efficiency without threatening their livelihood, sense of self-esteem, or sense of competence.

The Sounding Board essay could have been prescriptive for the efforts that need to be made to improve the quality of mental or behavioral health services for patients in primary care settings and the quality of primary care for the chronic and seriously mentally ill. Since managed care organizations are in the best position to shape practice behavior through financial incentives and penalties, these companies must be encouraged to emphasize high-quality *and* cost-efficient behavioral health care that is well integrated with general health care.

Academic departments of psychiatry and their primary care counterparts should attempt to secure their critical place in the managed care networks, to help define standards of care in those networks, and to incorporate their training programs into integrated care systems. Clinical delivery systems associated with academic health centers would require the cost-effective deployment of physicians, physician extenders, and a variety of mental health professionals across the span of care: from general and behavioral health screening to health promotion, counseling, and psychotherapy, as well as the prescription of medications (including psychotropic drugs) efficaciously. Optimally, the budget-based planning for a behavioral health product line (see Chapter 2) would include plans to integrate some of these services within academic primary care practice sites. In the context of improved patient satisfaction and outcome, the reasonable patient care costs of such an effort will need to be understood and borne by responsible managed care organizations.

Summary

The emphasis on primary care as the cornerstone of managed care confronts academic departments of psychiatry and their generalist counterparts with an age-old and significant challenge: the underdiagnosis and inadequate treatment of mental disorders and subthreshold conditions in primary care practice—and its counterpart in the poor quality of general health care received by patients with chronic mental illnesses. Most studies have simply confirmed the problems. The few studies that have actually addressed possible solutions have identified the need for a broadly based approach that integrates mental or behavioral health services more effectively into primary care practice. The challenges involve improvements in the clinical delivery system, the implementation of cross-disciplinary training programs, and the identification of the costs and cost savings that might result from better program integration. At this juncture, the evidence does not support the case for primary care physicians as mental health service providers—or of psychiatrists as primary care physicians to the chronically mentally ill—if patient outcome is the yardstick of quality of care.

Without significant changes in the delivery system and the skills and knowledge of the providers, arguments to include mental health care in primary care practice sound like political rhetoric without substance.

Enhanced screening efforts, by themselves, are simply not enough to deal with the problem. On the other hand, as noted by Sturm and Wells (1995) and by Katon et al. (1995, 1996), with adequate attention to quality improvement measures (and strong liaison, consultation, and some direct behavioral health services in the general health care milieu), the treatment of some mentally ill patients (i.e., those with major depressive disorder) can be cost-efficient in primary care settings. Because the delivery system is really not ready for rapid overhaul, the present situation constitutes a crisis for psychiatry as for primary care disciplines. The danger is that primary care disciplines will accept the responsibility for behavioral health services without a strong support system in place. The opportunity is for the present crisis to force academic psychiatry departments and their primary care counterparts to address long-standing problems in a manner that will strengthen their disciplines, their training programs, and the well-being of their patients.

References

Adams WL, Barry KL, Fleming MF: Screening for problem drinking in older primary care patients. JAMA 276:1964–1967, 1996

American Psychiatric Association: Diagnostic and Statistical Manual of Mental Disorders, 3rd Edition, Revised. Washington, DC, American Psychiatric Association, 1987

American Psychiatric Association: Diagnostic and Statistical Manual of Mental Disorders, 4th Edition. Washington, DC, American Psychiatric Association, 1995a

American Psychiatric Association: Diagnostic and Statistical Manual of Mental Disorders, 4th Edition—Primary Care Version (DSM-IV–PC). Washington, DC, American Psychiatric Association, 1995b

Babor TF, Grant M: From clinical research to secondary prevention: international collaboration in the development of the Alcohol Use Disorders Identification Test (AUDIT). Alcohol Health Res World 13:371–374, 1989

Barsky AJ, Borus JF: Somatization and medicalization in the era of managed care. JAMA 274:1931–1934, 1995

Block SD, Clark-Chiarelli N, Peters AS: Academia's chilly climate for primary care. JAMA 276:677–682, 1996

Bridges KW, Goldberg DP: Somatic presentation of DSM III psychiatric disorders in primary care. J Psychosom Res 29:563–569, 1985

Bryant E, Shimizu I: Sample design, sampling and estimation procedures for the National Ambulatory Medical Care Survey. Vital Health Stat 1988

Cartwright A: Patients and Their Doctors: A Study of General Practice. London, Routledge & Kegan Paul, 1967

deGruy F: Mental Health Care in the Primary Care Setting. Primary Care: America's Health in a New Era. Washington, DC, National Academy Press, 1996, Appendix D

Depression Guideline Panel: Depression in primary care, Vol 1: detection and diagnosis (AHCPR Publ No 93-0550). Rockville, MD, U.S. Department of Health and Human Services, 1993a

Depression Guideline Panel: Depression in primary care, Vol 2: treatment of major depression (AHCPR Publ No 93-0551). Rockville, MD, U.S. Department of Health and Human Services, 1993b

Donaldson M, Yordy K, Vanselow N: Defining Primary Care: An Interim Report. Washington, DC, Institute of Medicine, 1994, pp 1–38

Ewing JA: Detecting alcoholism: the CAGE questionnaire. JAMA 252:1905–1907, 1984

Fleming MF, Barry KL: A three-sample test of a masked alcohol screening questionnaire. Alcohol Alcohol 26:81–91, 1991

Garfield SR, Collen MF, Feldman R, et al: Evaluation of ambulatory medical care system. N Engl J Med 295:426–431, 1976

Greco PJ, Eisenberg JM: Changing physicians' practices. N Engl J Med 329:1271–1273, 1993

Hall RCW, Gardner ER, Popkin MK, et al: Unrecognized physical illness prompting psychiatric admission: a prospective study. Am J Psychiatry 138:629–635, 1981

Hays RD, Wells KB, Sherbourne DC, et al: Functioning and well-being outcomes of patients with depression compared with chronic general medical illnesses. Arch Gen Psychiatry 52:11–19, 1995

Henk HJ, Katzelnick DJ, Kobak KA, et al: Medical costs attributed to depression among patients with a history of high medical expenses in a health maintenance organization. Arch Gen Psychiatry 53:899–904, 1996

Higgins ES: A review of unrecognized mental illness in primary care: prevalence, natural history, and efforts to change the course. Arch Fam Med 3:908–917, 1994

Higgins ES: Obsessive-compulsive spectrum disorders in primary care: the possibilities and the pitfalls. J Clin Psychiatry 57(suppl 8):7–9, 1996

Hilkevitch A: Psychiatric disturbance in outpatients of a general medical outpatient clinic. International Journal of Neuropsychiatry 1:371–375, 1965

Howard KI, Cornille TA, Lyons JS, et al: Patterns of mental health service utilization. Arch Gen Psychiatry 53(suppl 8):696–703, 1996

Johnson JG, Spitzer RL, Williams JBW, et al: Psychiatric comorbidity, health status, and functional impairment associated with alcohol abuse/dependence in primary care patients: findings of the PRIME-MD 1000 study. Journal of Clinical and Consulting Psychology 63:133–140, 1995

Katon W: Panic disorder: relationship to high medical utilization, unexplained physical symptoms and medical costs. J Clin Psychiatry 57:1–17, 1996

Katon W, Von Korff M, Lin E, et al: Collaborative management to achieve treatment guidelines: impact on depression in primary care. JAMA 273:1026–1031, 1995

Katon W, Robinson P, Von Korff M, et al: A multifaceted intervention to improve treatment of depression in primary care. Arch Gen Psychiatry 53:924–932, 1996

Koran LM, Sox HC, Marton KI, et al: Medical evaluation of psychiatric patients. Arch Gen Psychiatry 46:733–740, 1989

Kroenke K, Spitzer RL, Williams JB, et al: Physical symptoms in primary care: predictors of psychiatric disorders and functional impairment. Arch Fam Med 3:774–779, 1994

Lipowski ZJ: Somatization: the concept and its clinical application. Am J Psychiatry 145:1358–1368, 1988

Maurer K: Primary care mental health screen; PRIME-MD gets mixed reviews in the medical field. Clinical Psychiatry News 23–24, 1996

Mayfield DG, McLeod G, Hall P: The CAGE questionnaire: validation of a new alcoholism screening instrument. Am J Psychiatry 131:1121–1123, 1974

McFarland BH, Freeborn DK, Mullooly JP, et al: Utilization patterns among long-term enrollees in a prepaid group practice health maintenance organization. Med Care 23:1221–1233, 1985

Meredith LS, Wells KB, Kaplan SH, et al: Counseling typically provided for depression: role of clinician specialty and payment system. Arch Gen Psychiatry 53:905–912, 1996

Olfson M, Broadhead WE, Weissman MM, et al: Subthreshold psychiatric symptoms in a primary care group practice. Arch Gen Psychiatry 53:880–886, 1996

Pincus HA, Strain JJ, Houpt JL, et al: Models of mental health training in primary care. JAMA 249:3065–3068, 1983

Pincus HA, Vettorello NE, McQueen LE, et al: Bridging the gap between psychiatry and primary care; the DSM-IV-PC. Psychosomatics 36:329–335, 1995

Pokorny AD, Miller BA, Kaplan HB: The brief MAST: a shortened version of the Michigan Alcoholism Screening Test. Am J Psychiatry 129:342–345, 1972

Regier DA, Goldberg ID, Taube CA: The defacto US mental health services system. Arch Gen Psychiatry 35:685–693, 1978

Rosenblatt RA: Identifying primary care disciplines by analyzing the diagnostic content of ambulatory care. J Am Board Fam Pract 8:41–44, 1995

Schulberg HC, Block MR, Madonia JJ, et al: Treating major depression in primary care practice: eight-month clinical outcomes. Arch Gen Psychiatry 53:913–919, 1996

Selzer ML: The Michigan Alcoholism Screening Test: the quest for a new diagnostic instrument. Am J Psychiatry 127:1653–1658, 1971

Selzer ML, Vinokur A, Van Rooijen L: A self-administered Short Michigan Alcoholism Screening Test (SMAST). J Stud Alcohol 36:117–126, 1975

Shapiro S, Skinner EA, Kessler LG, et al: Utilization of health and mental health services: three epidemiologic catchment area sites. Arch Gen Psychiatry 41:971–978, 1984

Sherbourne CD, Wells KB, Meredith LS: Comorbid anxiety disorder and the functioning and well-being of chronically ill patients of general medical providers. Arch Gen Psychiatry 53:889–895, 1996

Shore JH: Psychiatry at a crossroad: our role in primary care. Am J Psychiatry 153:1398–1399, 1996

Smith GR: The course of somatization and its effects on utilization of health care resources. Psychosomatics 35:263–267, 1994

Smith GR, Monson RP, Roy DC: Psychiatric consultation in somatization disorder: a randomized controlled study. N Engl J Med 314:1407–1423, 1986

Smith GR, Rost K, Kashner TM: A trial of the effect of standardized psychiatric consultation on health outcomes and costs in somatizing patients. Arch Gen Psychiatry 52:238–243, 1995

Sox HC Jr, Koran LM, Sox CH, et al: A medical algorithm for detecting physical disease in psychiatric patients. Journal of Hospital and Community Psychiatry 40:1270–1276, 1989

Spitzer RL, Williams JBW, Kroenke E, et al: Utility of a new procedure for diagnosing mental disorders in primary care: the PRIME-MD 1000 study. JAMA 272:1749–1756, 1994

Spitzer RL, Kroenke K, Linzer M, et al: Health-related quality of life in primary care patients with mental disorders: results from the PRIME-MD 1000 study. JAMA 274:1511–1517, 1995

Stewart AL, Greenfield S, Hays RD, et al: Functional status and well-being of patients with chronic conditions: results from the Medical Outcomes Study. JAMA 262:907–913, 1989

Strain JJ, Pincus HA, Gise LH, et al: The role of psychiatry in the training of primary care physicians. Gen Hosp Psychiatry 8:372–385, 1986

Sturm R, Wells KB: How can care for depression become more cost effective? JAMA 273:1026–1031, 1995

Swenson WM, Morese RM: The use of a Self-Administered Alcoholism Screening Test (SAAST) in a medical center. Mayo Clin Proc 50:204–208, 1975

Tiemens BG, Ormel J, Simon GE: Occurrence, recognition and outcome of psychological disorders in primary care. Am J Psychiatry 153(suppl 5):636–644, 1996

Wells KB, Stewart A, Hays RD, et al: The functioning and well-being of depressed patients: results from the Medical Outcomes Study. JAMA 262:914–919, 1989

CHAPTER 6

The Impact of Academic Psychiatry on the Mental Health Care of Veterans: A Fifty-Year Perspective

Thomas B. Horvath, M.D., F.R.A.C.P.

While a number of studies have explored the nature of the health care system of the Department of Veterans Affairs (Veterans Health Administration, or VHA) and its relationship to academic medicine (Association of- American Medical Colleges 1990; Alexander 1992; Fisher and Welch 1995; Gronvall 1989; Hollingsworth and Bondy 1990; Iglehart 1985, 1996), the evolution of the mental health delivery system of the Veterans Administration (VA) and its relationship to academic psychiatry has not been given equivalent attention (Errera 1988, 1992). Yet the mental health units of the VA treat more than half a million patients a year, employ over 1,600 psychiatrists, train over 800 residents, and help to generate over $50 million per year in research funds.

For decades, VA medical centers were the reliable, although not glamorous, junior partners in the academic enterprise. Since the early 1980s, a decade and a half of straight-line budgets have taken their toll on the quality of this partnership, and the press has raised questions about the quality of VA care. A strong and predictable relationship between academia and the VA could no longer be taken for granted (Froelicher 1996; Schafer 1996). The failure of the Clinton plan for health care reform (Skocpol 1996) triggered an identity crisis in the VA. Was the VA to become a potential participant in the marketplace competition between managed care organizations or was it to become a tired, bureaucratic government entity that had outlived its usefulness? Were VHA medical centers akin to academic health care centers, sought out for their expert care, research, and teaching, or were they more like the state hospitals of old, places of asylum for patients nobody else wanted?

In 1993, Secretary Brown, a combat-injured Vietnam veteran and a relentless advocate of veterans affairs (Brown 1993), appointed Ken Kizer, M.D., a public health– and environmental medicine–trained Navy veteran (and a former director of health for the state of California) as undersecretary for VHA to try to answer these questions. Dr. Kizer has been able to focus the anxieties and energies generated by the VHA's internal problems and turbulent external relationships and has embarked the VA's Department of Medicine and Surgery on a process of reform (Kizer 1995, 1996a). Some observers liken this attempt to the major reorganization of the VA 50 years ago that created the Department of Medicine and Surgery (DMS, the old name for VHA) and that brought medical schools into partnerships with VA hospitals according to the famous Policy Memorandum No. 2, issued on January 30, 1946, quoted in Association of American Medical Colleges (1990).

Historical Roots

The VA system was born in the aftermath of the Civil War (Adkins 1967). Nothing prepared Americans for the size, scope, and brutality of that war, its high levels of mortality and physical morbidity, and its massive dislocation of the lives and permanent careers of tens of thousands of young men. Many returning soldiers were unfit for regular occupations or for settled modes of life. There were high levels of iatrogenic opiate addiction among the recovered wounded, and DaCosta's "irritable heart syndrome" and Weir Mitchell's "exhaustion" probably contributed to their social disabilities in a manner entirely similar to the role of posttraumatic stress disorder (PTSD) and substance abuse in the lives of Vietnam veterans.

The Union soon established veterans homes and domiciliaries (some of which now form the nucleus of our oldest VA medical centers). These facilities were military-style lodgings, with benign regimentation and attempts at resocialization and rehabilitation. Their philosophy was similar to the moral treatment practiced in the progressive mental hospitals of the earlier part of the century. In the VA domiciliary however, the rehabilitative, moral approach has persisted and now forms part of the foundation for contemporary work therapy and residential rehabilitation. As the main veteran service organization (VSO) of the era, the Grand Army of the Republic reached the height of its influence some 30 years after the Civil War, successfully lobbying for veteran pensions, expansion of the domiciliaries, and other preferential treatment for veterans. The timing of its role was very similar to the VSOs of today. Skocpol (1992) has described these beginnings of formal social policy in this country in aiding soldiers and mothers.

In 1930 the various bureaus dealing with veterans were brought together into one agency, the Veterans Administration. General Edward Hines, an incorruptible but conservative and highly cost-conscious Republican, became its administrator (Adkins 1967). He was a good bureaucrat and civil servant who believed in "systems" and sound management. He was very protective of his charges, the veteran inmates, and the staff looking after them. Veterans were expected to accept the discipline of the institutions, and the staff members were expected to accept the rules of civil service. Patient self-determination and professional independence were both anathema to the VA. In some ways, the system felt more comfortable in isolation. VA hospitals for tuberculosis were built in the sparsely populated Southwest. Neuropsychiatric hospitals were built in country areas, with the requisite 400 acres for horticultural therapy. General Hines strongly (and successfully) disagreed with his critics, who objected to the segregation of veterans into self-contained, distant compounds.

General Hines dealt with physicians and nurses in an equally paternalistic manner. Aspiring clinical professionals had to be appointed by a cumbersome civil service process. While the general and most other VA managers respected the clinical skills of professionals, they did not perceive them as good candidates for organizational leadership. Nor were they granted any structures of self-governance. As early as 1924, there were attempts to establish a professionally independent Medical Corps in the VA, and over the next two decades, General Hines successfully resisted 24 different congressional initiatives to set up a Department of Medicine and Surgery that would have produced some professional independence from the bureaucracy. He was equally resistant to the approaches by some medical schools in the early 1940s to develop relationships with the VA.

Hines was a good manager whose 22-year administration was marked by an increase in bed capacity (from 15,000 to 81,000) and an increase in the number of facilities (from 45 to 97). Yet the VA was perceived by many as a complacent and inflexible organization, whose medical care was mediocre and separated by physical distance and bureaucratic attitudes from mainstream medicine. The system cracked under the stress of World War II and performed very poorly (compared to military medicine). In the European theater of operations, General Paul Hawley, M.D., established a system in which a medical school would sponsor a military hospital and supply much of its staff. Thus military medicine was able to rapidly adapt the technological advances and logistic improvements developed in academia to its own needs. For instance, some military psychiatrists rediscovered Thomas Salmon's work on crisis intervention during the World War I and successfully returned combat-stressed men to duty. Yet other veterans with combat stress, not fortunate to be treated by military psychiatrists from academia, ended up on hospital ships with a diagnosis of psychosis and were consigned to neuropsychiatric VA facilities to be institutionalized for years.

The physically injured did not fare much better in a VA that was also stripped of its best staff by the needs of the military. Not surprisingly, in late 1944 there were a series of exposés in the press. These reports triggered a flurry of investigations, which minimized the problems but failed to restore the confidence of the public in the VA. President Truman replaced General Hines with General Omar Bradley, a leader known for his care and compassion for his troops. Bradley had worked closely with Hawley in Europe and respected him for his professionalism and his spirit of innovation. Thus Hawley became the first chief medical director of the DMS of the VA; he in turn appointed Dr. Paul Magnuson, an academic orthopedic surgeon, as the director of academic relationships. Under their leadership, physicians and nurses were hired outside civil service rules. Affiliations were developed with medical schools, and new hospitals were built close to universities. A remarkable spirit of innovation invaded the VA, overcoming bureaucratic inertia (Magnuson 1960).

Psychiatry in the VA

Unfortunately, psychiatry failed to participate fully in this great reorganization of the VA. Initially the mental health activities of the VA were focused on the 50 or so neuropsychiatric hospitals that were located in the country or distant suburbs. Medical schools were not interested in these facilities unless they could be converted into general medical-surgical hospitals. Furthermore, in the postwar years, academic departments of psychiatry were psychoanalytic in their orientation, and the chronic psychotic population of VA hospitals did not appeal to them. Medicine and surgery dominated the highly affiliated VA teaching hospitals, and psychiatry was their junior partner. In one of the ironies of history, military and VA psychiatry, which had discovered the principles of crisis intervention and ambulatory treatment for combat stress reactions in World War II, promptly forgot them. The VA's mental health system settled into a comfortable, long-term institutional mode. Only modest innovations were introduced. The VA opened mental hygiene clinics to treat "neurotic" patients, established day treatment programs for ambulatory psychotics, and introduced new treatment modalities: electroconvulsive therapy (ECT), insulin coma, and pharmacotherapy.

Mental health was an early participant in the VA's cooperative studies program, where one of the first multisite studies of neuroleptic treatment of schizophrenia was carried out. Psychiatry continued to use the cooperative studies program, along with its infrastructure of core statistical and clinical trials support and its ability to initiate studies at numerous sites. The VA maintained its leadership in multisite clinical trials, including early studies on prefrontal lobotomy, chlorpromazine and other neuroleptics, antidepressants, alcohol withdrawal treatment, L-α-acetylmethadol (LAAM), methadone, lithium, and antabuse (Department of Veterans Affairs 1993b). Some of the better staffed, more progressive neuropsychiatric hospitals engaged in the community psychiatry movement of the early 1960s and developed innovative programs of work-related rehabilitation and residential care. Unfortunately, these social experiments were not widely publicized and did not regularly find their way into the literature.

The next wave of reform for academic psychiatry in the VA occurred when younger, more scientifically trained psychiatrists started to take over the chairmanships of major departments. The focus of American psychiatry shifted from psychoanalysis to descriptive diagnosis, biological research, and the formal evaluation of psychotherapies and social interventions. The relatively slow pace of the VA, the availability of beds for research, and the generous research support provided by the VA all made academic affiliations in psychiatry attractive (Department of Veterans Affairs 1993a). However, several problems continued to mar the full flowering of these relationships.

The distance between neuropsychiatric hospitals and medical schools was one issue. This difficulty was partially overcome by developing university-affiliated general psychiatry units in medical-surgical VA teaching hospitals or by moving new medical schools to the VA hospital campus. Philadelphia VA and the University of Pennsylvania, the Bronx VA and Mount Sinai, West Haven VA and Yale, and Portland VA and Oregon Health Sciences are examples of the first approach. As examples of the second approach, the Northport VA was the initial host to SUNY–Stony Brook, and North Chicago was essential to the development of the Chicago Medical School. In some particularly strong affiliations, the medical school embraced an entire VA campus, sometimes allowing the VA to build on university property (Stanford at Palo Alto) or expanding the VA facility in proximity to the university campus (the University of California–Los Angeles and the Brentwood and Wadsworth VAs).

The second problem was the dominance of medical specialties in the upper hierarchies of the VA, both in the Veterans Administration Central Office and in the field. However, when a dynamic dean, an enlightened chief of staff, and a committed chair of psychiatry saw the advantages of academic affiliations in psychiatry, these hierarchical turf problems could be resolved.

The third, more insidious problem was the Vietnam War and the social dislocations it caused. Veterans returning from Southeast Asia were not greeted with open arms, and their reception in the VA was distinctly chilly. Many young clinicians in the VA were antiwar or avoided war zone service through graduate school deferment, U.S. Public Health Services (USPHS) work, and so on. The VSOs were dominated by World War II veterans who were disturbed by the behavior of the younger veterans. The VA professionals did not recognize PTSD, and the VSOs did not want to admit its existence. Academic psychiatry in the VA saw in Vietnam veterans a source of disturbance of the emerging equilibrium, a distraction from steady teaching and research tasks. The presenting symptoms of substance abuse and "character disorder" were easier to focus on. The Nixon Administration did so and declared the first war on drugs.

The substance abuse treatment programs of the VA, already growing to deal with the alcohol problems of older veterans, now received a healthy infusion of new funds. Separate alcohol and drug dependence units were set up, the former to deal with middle-aged, middle-class veterans and the latter to deal with Vietnam veterans and with inner-city drug users. In a number of locations, the expansion of the treatment system was guided by academic medicine and psychiatry, and several centers of excellence were developed (Philadelphia VA, Bronx VA). In other hospitals, the substance abuse program dollars and full-time employee equivalents (FTEEs) were "raided" by medical administration and used for other clinical purposes.

Vietnam veterans felt alienated from the VA and failed to get attention from psychiatry for their psychological problems. They and their advocates (including Vietnam Veterans Against the War and Vietnam Veterans of America) turned to alternative systems of delivery. Rap groups, self-help systems, and peer counseling became the focus of attention. During the Carter Administration, a triple-amputee Vietnam veteran, Max Cleland, became the VA administrator. During his tenure, the VA finally recognized combat stress and the resulting PTSD as a valid, compensable disorder, and a community-based service delivery system of readjustment counseling centers or "vet centers" was set up (Senate Veterans Affairs Committee 1993). The advocates did not trust either the VA's institutional psychiatry or academic psychiatry to deliver these services. The vet centers moved away from medical centers into storefronts and other community locations. They were staffed mostly by peer counselors, social workers, and psychologists, most of whom were veterans and many of whom saw active combat in Vietnam. An alternative, nonbureaucratic VA came into existence, and academic psychiatry lost the opportunity to take a lead in the social transformation of the VA or to study the complex biopsychology of PTSD.

Psychiatry in the VA in the early 1980s was faced with an unaccomplished agenda. It had paid little attention to the raison d'être of the VA, combat stress disorder. With some notable exceptions, it failed to take advantage of the growth in substance abuse funding. It was unable to reform the delivery system for the chronically mentally ill. To its credit, it refused and resisted attempts at inappropriate deinstitutionalization (but at the cost of maintaining large and increasingly out-of-date inpatient facilities). Despite a huge investment in beds, the VA was confronted by the embarrassing statistic of over 200,000 veterans homeless on the streets of major cities. Finally, the growth in psychiatric research and education stalled during the budget cuts of the 1980s, and psychiatry appeared to be relegated to a permanent second-class citizenship (Senate Veterans Affairs Committee 1993).

A Yale professor, the chief of psychiatry at West Haven VA, was induced to move to Washington to become the director of Mental Health and Behavioral Sciences Service (Errera 1988, 1992). Through a combination of persuasiveness, bureaucratic politics, and calculated appeals to the "better side of our nature," he managed to garner special funding for all of these unfinished projects. He assembled an excellent team of professionals with academic backgrounds in Washington and in intellectual support centers at several Veterans Affairs Medical Centers (VAMCs) in close collaboration with their Medical Schools: West Haven, Palo Alto, White River Junction, Salt Lake City, and Ann Arbor. The new clinical programs for PTSD (Fontana et al. 1996), homelessness (Frisman et al. 1996), substance abuse (Moos 1996a,b), and serious mental illness (Special Committee for Seriously Mentally Ill Veterans 1995, 1997) were carefully and scientifically monitored.

The Mental Health of Veterans and the VA

There are 27 million veterans, of whom nearly 10% have service-related disabilities and nearly 6% are poor. Under the current eligibility rules, 8 million veterans can use the VA and nearly 3 million do so on an annual basis. The lifetime incidence of mental and addictive disorders among veterans is 5 million, of whom a little over 2 million would be currently eligible for VA care. Most of the mental disorders that the VA treats are chronic: characterized by remissions and exacerbation rather than definitive cures. Also, many veterans suffer from more than one mental disorder concurrently, most commonly an association of an alcohol or other substance abuse disorder with a major psychiatric disorder such as schizophrenia or PTSD. In addition, many veterans have medical problems (e.g., cardiac or pulmonary disease) as well.

Mental health services are integrated into the VA's network of 171 hospitals, 313 clinics, 123 nursing homes, 37 domiciliaries, and 202 vet centers. VHA employs over 200,000 people, and the overall health care budget is $16 billion, of which $2 billion goes for mental health. VHA employs 1,600 psychiatrists and 1,500 psychologists in mental health services. Veterans affairs health care centers (combinations of hospitals, clinics, nursing homes, and domiciliaries) vary much in size and complexity, but they are all Joint Commission–approved, and their average score is 5 to 10 points higher than that of comparable private-sector hospitals.

Consumers with mental and addictive disorders represent a sizable group of the veterans who use the VA. In 1995 the VHA treated 557,000 for mental disorders, including substance abuse, an increase of 12% since 1990. Of these, 68,000 needed inpatient care (and were admitted 1.5 times per year for an average length of stay of 24 days) and 494,000 received outpatient care, with an average of 13 visits per year. On a given working day, there are 12,000 veterans in psychiatric inpatient care, and another 26,000 are participating in outpatient care. VHA has shifted care to the ambulatory arena, increased outpatient visits, and reduced inpatient days during an overall increase in enrollment. Sociodemographic factors and distance from providers explain 44% of the variance in utilization: poor veterans in proximity to the VA center or clinic use its services (Rosenheck 1996).

Department of Veterans Affairs (DVA) mental health care programs are coordinated by the mental health and behavioral sciences strategic health group. It is the goal of this strategic health group to provide a continuum of care for veterans suffering from mental disorders, from the most intensive inpatient treatment units to innovative outpatient programs designed to maintain chronically ill patients in their communities and to do so cost-effectively. The mental health group also has responsibility for the policy direction of four special emphasis programs (for PTSD, homelessness, substance abuse, and serious mental illness) and for the generation and dissemination of new knowledge about the mental health of veterans.

Posttraumatic Stress Disorder

The VA has finally organized a comprehensive treatment system for combat-related PTSD. Vietnam veterans who once shunned the VA now are entering at rates comparable to veterans of other eras. PTSD workloads have been increasing as PTSD services have expanded. In fiscal year (FY) 1991, 37,393 unique veterans were treated, 10,087 of these in inpatient services; in FY 1993, 49,915 were treated, 11,610 in inpatient services. It is anticipated that these increases in PTSD workload will continue, since almost half a million Vietnam veterans may still have untreated PTSD.

The National Vietnam Veterans Readjustment Study found that African-American and Hispanic veterans suffered from PTSD at a disproportionately high rate compared to their white counterparts. Specifically, the prevalence of PTSD was 27.9% among Hispanics, 20.6% among African-Americans, and 13.7% among whites or others. The Vietnam Veterans Project (Matsunaga Study) is now looking at PTSD among Vietnam veterans of Asian, Pacific Islander, Native American, and Native Alaskan descent. The needs of minority veterans who suffer from PTSD can be addressed by better understanding the scope of the problem and by developing ethnoculturally sensitive assessment and treatment procedures. There is a significant opportunity here for culturally competent academic psychiatrists.

Homelessness

There are probably 200,000 veterans homeless at a given time. About 50% of homeless veterans have substance abuse disorders, and 40% suffer from serious mental illnesses. In addition, 44% of homeless veterans have serious medical problems. The VA has developed an impressive constellation of programs for homeless veterans, and these programs constitute the largest integrated network of programs to assist homeless individuals in the nation. Although each treatment program is tailored to meet the needs of homeless veterans in a given location, these programs have common characteristics that include aggressive outreach, assessment of clinical needs, medical and mental health treatment, case management, and placement in contract community-based residential care facilities or admission to the VA's own domiciliary care programs for biopsychosocial rehabilitation.

The VA has developed partnerships with federal, state, and community programs in order to expand and enhance the range of services that can be offered to homeless veterans. The VA's partnership with the Social Security Administration has led to expedited claims processing for homeless veterans eligible for Social Security benefits. The VA's partnership with HUD has led to an effective program that links VA case management services with dedicated Section 8 rental assistance vouchers. The VA's coordination with community service providers is equally important. Some of the most effective collaborations take place between VA's homeless programs and VSOs. There is great scope for social anthropological and health services research in the area of homelessness.

Addictive Disorders

As many as a third of all veterans seeking care from the VA have alcohol and, less frequently, drug use disorders. Since the establishment of the initial substance abuse treatment programs in the 1960s, the VA's treatment capability has undergone significant expansion. The VA now operates substance abuse treatment programs at 159 of its medical centers and outpatient clinics. In FY 1995, inpatient rehabilitation programs treated more than 55,000 veterans. Over 40,000 of these patients had a primary or associated drug abuse disorder, with the balance treated for problems related to alcohol abuse alone. In addition to those veterans seen on specialized units, another 31,000 patients with addictive disorders received care on VA general psychiatry units and 40,000 on VA medical and surgical units. VA substance abuse outpatient programs have treated over 108,000 veterans in almost 1.9 million visits.

In FY 1980, the VA was given authority to contract with non-VA community halfway houses for rehabilitation services for veterans with substance abuse disorders. In a given year this program supports nearly 6,000 veterans in an estimated 300 community halfway house for 60 to 90 days of care.

The VA addictive disorders treatment system is a unique and highly vulnerable treatment, educational, and research resource, for both veterans and the nation as a whole. The integrity of any one aspect is dependent on the integrity of the others. For instance, large-scale outcome studies on treatment are probably best performed in the VA because of the large number of patients available and because long-term follow-up is facilitated (patients tend to remain in the system).

Erosion of the substance abuse treatment capability, as has occurred in the past when national attention has turned away from substance abuse issues, affects both research and training. From a purely clinical perspective, substance abuse remains a leading health problem among veterans. Most veterans with addictive disorders do not receive treatment for this problem. Substance abuse is a routine finding among homeless veterans and is probably the major cause of homelessness in a significant cohort, it is ubiquitous among veterans with PTSD, and it has a major impact on the utilization of medical and surgical resources in the VA.

Serious Mental Illness

Beginning with the establishment of an array of outpatient programs in the 1960s, the VA has been an innovator in mental health care delivery. Day hospitals provided time-limited, intensive care to avoid hospitalization or transition back into community living. Day treatment centers provided extended supportive care for chronically mentally ill patients, decreasing hospitalizations and improving their quality of life. Community-based residential treatment centers have decreased inpatient stays and facilitated the recovery of veterans. Collaborative arrangements with local residential care providers and the development of compensated work therapy or therapeutic housing programs have added a strong rehabilitative dimension. A special congressionally chartered committee now monitors the developments in this area (Special Committee for Seriously Mentally Ill Veterans 1995, 1997).

Despite the fact that outpatient and off-site or community-based psychiatric care is often more appropriate than inpatient psychiatric care, only about 25% of the VA's mental health budget goes to outpatient services, well under the 38% average for outpatient expenditures by state mental health agencies. Patients with serious chronic mental illnesses such as schizophrenia are rarely resolved, and relapses will occur without good follow-up. New studies show that almost three-quarters of VA schizophrenia patients and two-thirds of alcohol abuse patients are still using VA health services 6–10 years later. Such studies would argue for a strong support of ambulatory services, supported by an effective health services research and evaluation component.

Mental Health Research

To maintain and enhance the quality of care provided to veterans suffering from mental disorders, the linkage of clinical services with education and research is essential. Innovations in clinical care, not only in the biological aspects of psychiatric diagnosis and treatment but also in terms of psychosocial therapies, must be available to VA patients. The VA is a leader in many areas of mental health research (e.g., PTSD, schizophrenia, and alcohol or substance abuse), and the benefits are directly applied to our patients (Department of Veterans Affairs 1993a). An academic environment also serves to attract and retain high-quality clinicians in VA treatment settings. Several reports reviewed by the commission on the future structure of VA (1991) have indicated, however, that more resources should be made available to VA mental health research. Kety pointed out a decade ago that less than 10% of VA research resources were directed to mental health research, while over 40% of all VA bed days of care were provided to veterans suffering from mental disorders. Psychiatric patients now account for 33% of all VA inpatients at any time and 43% of total inpatient days of care, and 22% of all VA users are in mental health treatment. Yet the percentage of VA research funding for mental health has only increased to about 12% of the total research budget since Kety's original report, or Detre's follow-up in 1990.

Of the $50 million generated by mental health research, the VA research and development service accounts for $25 million; research projects by VA psychiatric researchers are funded by non-VA sources for another $25 million. The indirect research support ("release time") given to mental health is only about half of what is provided for medicine on a per capita and per earned dollar basis.

Most VA research support is awarded to individual physician principal investigators through the VA's research service (although there are three schizophrenia biological research center grants and three alcohol centers). VA research funds are awarded on the basis of the quality of proposed studies to individual researchers, who conceptualize, design, and carry out funded studies (Department of Veterans Affairs 1993b). The VA also has a health services research and development (HSR&D) program. The HSR&D program was established to investigate factors related to the organization, delivery, costs, and outcomes of VA health care programs. Three of the nine HSR&D centers have a mental health focus.

At least in part, the lower rate of psychiatric research funding is a function of the high clinical workloads of VA psychiatrists and psychologists, which limits the time they can devote to research (Senate Veterans Affairs Committee 1993). In academic settings, most attending physicians in medicine have major clinical responsibilities for only several months a year, whereas most psychiatrists, due to the clinical necessity of maintaining ongoing relationships with their patients and because of low staffing levels, must devote all working time to their inpatient unit or clinic work. To begin to correct those imbalances, the concept of mental illness research, education, and clinical care centers (MIRECCs) has been discussed and suggested in legislation (Senate Veterans Affairs Committee 1993). Modeled after the successful geriatric research, education, and clinical care centers (GRECCs), proposals have been made for the creation of five MIRECCs across the VA health care system, located in VA facilities with established psychiatry and psychology training programs. Finally, in 1996, recurrent funding for MIRECCs was authorized in Public Law 104-226. Given the importance of health care delivery and outcomes research for improving care to veterans, the legislation focuses the MIRECC in this area. The first two MIRECCs were funded in July 1997. It is hoped that they will replicate the success of the PTSD research center, which provides a model for integrating different research and clinical approaches, a central problem of the VA.

Public Law 98-528 mandated the establishment of a VA National Center for PTSD to carry out a broad range of multidisciplinary activities in research, education, and training. The National Center, established in 1989, is a consortium that currently is comprised of six sites (National Center for Posttraumatic Stress Disorder 1995). The executive division, located at White River Junction VAMC, carries out strategic planning and directs the overall operations of the National Center and collaborates closely with Dartmouth. It houses the PTSD resource center, which has established a comprehensive bibliographic database on PTSD. The behavioral sciences division at the Boston VAMC and Boston University develops scientifically validated instruments to measure PTSD. The clinical neuroscience division at VAMC West Haven and Yale is one of the few sites in the world investigating the effects of severe stress on brain function and developing new biological approaches for the diagnosis and treatment of PTSD. The clinical laboratory and education division, at the Menlo Park VAMC, with some Stanford connections, serves as a major site for research protocols, sleep studies, cross-cultural investigations, and educational activities. A women's health sciences division, located at VAMC Boston, was added to the consortium in 1993. It focuses on research and education on the psychological and biological impact of military service on women. The Pacific center for PTSD, created in 1992, focuses on cross-cultural issues. The Northeast program evaluation center at VAMC West Haven, which carries the ongoing evaluation of all PTSD and homeless programs, is also programmatically linked to the National Center.

Another area of National Center activity has focused on major national and world events such as human-caused and natural disasters: the Loma Prieta earthquake in 1989, Hurricane Andrew in 1992, the 1991 hostage crisis in Iraq and Kuwait, the Persian Gulf War, and various peacekeeping and humanitarian missions. These disasters have fostered collaborative activities between the VA's National Center for PTSD, the Red Cross, the Federal Emergency Management Agency, and other cabinet-level departments such as defense, state, health and human services, transportation, and commerce. Such collaborations have led to unprecedented opportunities to study the emotional sequelae of war and disasters immediately after the experience and to provide needed clinical interventions close enough in time to the original trauma that there is hope of avoiding the chronicity and comorbidities common to PTSD.

The Future

During the deliberations on the Clinton Administration's health care reform, the VA was assured a firm place in the emerging system. The VA would have expanded its scope and seriously entertained notions of providing care for dependents, similar to the military health care system. The role of medical schools and affiliations was reconfirmed. The failure of the Clinton plan, while disappointing, did not mean the cessation of reform activity within the VA. Reforms were badly needed. In the early 1990s several press exposés and Inspector General and General Accounting Office investigations raised serious questions about the quality and efficiency of the VA system (Commission on the Future Structure of Veterans Health Care 1991).

Unfortunately, large infusions of money were not available to solve these problems (General Accounting Office 1996b). Nor was there an atmosphere congenial to dramatic increases in central federal interventions, as there was during the first major reorganization of the VA under General Omar Bradley. Help was not offered from the academic community, because academic health centers themselves were reeling from the onslaughts of managed care. Nevertheless, the reorganization had a number of similarities to its first reorganization 50 years earlier. Secretary Brown, through his experience as a disabled American veteran, shared with Omar Bradley a commitment to the welfare of GIs. The chief medical directors, Drs. Hawley and Kizer, also shared certain traits: both were physicians, both were veterans, and both had successfully managed large systems (the European Theater of Operations (ETO) in Europe in the 1940s and California's health system in the 1980s).

Neither was bound by the bureaucratic traditions and old perceptions of the VA. While the atmosphere of the government was entirely different in the two eras, the leaders of the VA successfully aligned themselves with the prevailing attitudes and rode popular sentiments. In the aftermath of World War II this sentiment was a belief in the legacy of successful big government and in partnerships with educational institutions. In the mid 1990s the prevailing notion was the idea of reinventing the government to make it lean and responsive to consumer demands. The principles of VHA's reorganization, enumerated by Kizer (1995), bear these marks of government reinvention (General Accounting Office 1996a):

> In addition to a Departmental commitment to improving the quality of veterans health care, other factors are prompting change within VHA. Chief among these is the profound change in the way health care is being provided in the United States. Technological advances, economic factors, demographic changes and the rise of managed health care, among other things, are causing a dramatic shift away from inpatient care and a corresponding increase in ambulatory care. VHA needs to adapt its service delivery to align with the changes occurring in the larger health care environment.

President Clinton's initiative to reinvent and streamline government also mandates that VHA examine its organizational practices and become a more agile and cost-efficient health care delivery system (General Accounting Office 1996a,b).

Further, in recent years, numerous government and nongovernment reports have consistently concluded that fundamental changes are needed in the health care system (including VHA) to make it more patient responsive and efficient (Charns and Tewksbury 1993; Commission on the Future Structure of Veterans Health Care 1991). Among the principal changes that have been recommended for VHA are

- Restructuring the operational structure of VHA.
- Redistributing VHA health care resources to better meet veterans' needs.

■ Using innovative approaches to improve veterans' access to VHA health care.

■ Decentralization of decision making and operations.

The resulting "new VA" should (Kizer 1996b)

■ Increase ambulatory care access points.

■ Emphasize primary care.

■ Integrate the delivery assets to provide an interdependent, interlacing system of care.

This restructuring includes a new distribution of VHA headquarters and field responsibilities. Headquarters' purview includes the development of systemwide policies, clinical protocols, and critical pathways; definition of expected levels of performance; and monitoring of outcomes. Implementation of policies and control of processes, operations, and decision making are vested with the field. The authority and responsibility to accomplish these functions is similarly given to the field leadership, who are held accountable for meeting defined levels of patient satisfaction, access, quality, and efficiency.

The new field organization is based on coordinating and integrating VHA's health care delivery assets into 22 veterans integrated service networks (VISN). The VISN structure is derived from a model of organizational management that emphasizes quality patient care, customer satisfaction, innovation, personal initiative, and accountability (Charns and Tewksbury 1993). The basic budgetary and planning unit of health care delivery shifts from individual medical centers to the integrated service networks providing for populations of veteran beneficiaries in defined geographic areas. These network service areas and their veteran populations are defined on the basis of VHA's natural patient referral patterns; aggregate numbers of beneficiaries and facilities needed to support and provide primary, secondary, and tertiary care; and, to a lesser extent, political jurisdictional boundaries such as state borders.

As an integrated system of care, the VISN model will optimally promote a pooling of resources and an expansion of community-based access points for primary care. In this scheme, the hospital will remain an important, albeit less central, component of a larger, more coordinated community-based network of care. In such a system, emphasis is placed on the integration of ambulatory care and acute and extended inpatient services so as to provide a coordinated continuum of care, often across the network. Mental health is emerging as such an integrated service line in most of the networks. Furthermore, closer collaboration between mental health and primary care is developing along two models. In the first, a traditional liaison model, mental health practitioners move into general internal medicine clinics to practice, teach, and conduct research. In the other, a mental health primary care model, psychiatrists assisted by physician assistants and nurse practitioners assume responsibility for the comprehensive care management of patients and involve internists only as consultants. New curricula are being developed for residency training as well.

In order to provide excellence in education and research, certain guiding principles have been enumerated (Kizer 1996a):

- Education and research activities should be held accountable to, and managed with, performance expectations and outcome measures in the same manner as clinical care.
- The VA's educational offerings and research effects should emphasize areas of greatest societal need as well as greatest need of veterans.
- Academic affiliation agreements should be fair and equitable, and VA personnel should have recognition and influence in affiliated universities commensurate with the contributions of their educational and research services.

To implement the restructuring of affiliate relationships, two major policy committees have published detailed reports: one chaired by Dr. Robert Petersdorf, former president of the American Association of Medical Colleges (AAMC), on residency training and one by Dr. George Rutherford from the University of California–Berkeley on research realignment. These reports provide specific details about implementing these principles (Petersdorf 1996).

What is clear from reading these reports is that unlike many managed care organizations, the VA is still willing to partner with academic health care centers to fulfill the basic principles of the VA's mission. Thus, the current reorganization of VHA should maintain the VA's his-

toric commitment to patient care, teaching, and research—the acquisition and dissemination of new knowledge in the service of veterans'
health. If we are to learn from the history of the earlier affiliations, we
should deal better with some of the historic tensions that prevented
VHA from reaching its full potential, especially in mental health, during
the first 50 years of its existence, and we should more fully exploit the
strategic alliances that helped it to survive.

Summary

This historic overview of the VA health care system describes recurring
themes and tensions between the VA and academia and within the VA.
The first tension to develop and persist was that between clinicians and
administrators (Magnuson 1960). Clinicians come from the independent
learned professions and often deal poorly with administrators who have
an organizational and bureaucratic mind set. At least part of the solution
should be to encourage more clinicians to obtain managerial and leadership training while maintaining their direct involvement with patient
care. In turn, more administrators should do part of their training in
clinical departments, and the two groups should have joint educational
and work experiences. The emergence of patient-centered care and service or product lines, the ongoing support of leadership training courses
in the VA, and the reduced bureaucratization expected from the "reinventing the government" movement are all positive signs pointing toward
a more integrated approach.

The second tension, and a major contributor to psychiatry's problems, has been the conflict between clinicians and academics (Alexander
1992). Not only did academic psychiatry fail to influence many psychiatrists and many of the neuropsychiatric hospitals, but it also failed to
give an academic role to most psychologists, social workers, and psychiatric nurses. Common teaching functions and exercises should be
encouraged. Most VA clinicians enjoy teaching, and the VA's role in this
part of academic life is rarely controversial. Academic investigators on
the other side are increasingly sensitive to the application of their work
to clinical situations, and the approach of bringing science from the
bench to the bedside is gaining more support. Departments could ex-

periment with team teaching, using scientists and clinicians in tandem. The reorganization of affiliations is going to bring these issues into sharper focus. Departments not willing to engage in new ways of relating clinical and research work, and unwilling to invest in teaching or disrespecting their VA staff, may well find their role diminish in a network while other, more flexible, departments benefit.

The third tension that soured the atmosphere during the Vietnam War was the relationship between clinicians and veterans. Clinicians often failed to appreciate the importance of war zone service to veterans (Rosenheck and Massari 1993). The lack of military experience of most VA mental health staff added to the usual tensions between mental health providers and consumers. The rise of a consumer movement, friendly to research (e.g., National Alliance for the Mentally Ill (NAMI) and National Mental Health Association) and open to collaboration with Veterans Service Organizations (VSOs), should help to some extent. The VA is also making more efforts to hear from its consumers through advisory councils and customer surveys. Recruitment of staff with active duty or reservist experience should further improve the level of empathy toward specific veterans' issues. VSOs are also becoming more aware and more supportive of mental health issues, especially in the areas of PTSD, substance abuse, and family problems.

However, these persistent but reducible tensions do not typify the entire VA-academic experience. A very positive alliance has grown up between congressional staffers, central office personnel, and VSO officers, which has helped on numerous occasions to protect VA programs and develop new initiatives. People often moved around the apices of this "iron triangle." Their relationships with one another and their common goals often led to a remarkable executive branch–legislative branch synchrony and equally remarkable feats of bipartisan working efforts. More recently, the waning of veteran membership in Congress and the reduction in bipartisan, amicable working groups has endangered this alliance.

Academic health care centers can help to restore the cooperation. By showing how academic institutions benefit veterans and in turn benefit the VA, they can broaden their legislative appeal. However, decentralization and reorganization also mean that more attention needs to be paid to local staff in the VA networks, in local congressional officers and to state and county legislators, and to VSO leaders in their state-level organizations. Academic institutions should be represented in the management assistance councils for the networks. Academic staff should get to know the participants in this "iron triangle"; their acquaintances will help them in VA and in general academic endeavors.

In some ways the challenges posed by the chronic illness of psychiatric patients represents an opportunity for academic psychiatry to demonstrate to the federal sector how to highlight quality as well as cost-effective management. For this approach to work, the VA system also needs to continue to incorporate research and innovation into mental illness treatment. This academic affiliation strategy still represents the best hope for the future of the VA's mental illness and psychiatric treatment delivery system and the best hope for veterans afflicted by mental and addictive disorders. The continued success of this partnership may also provide one model for the relationship between managed care organizations and academic health care centers.

References

Adkins RE: Medical care of veterans (Committee Print No. 4, 90th Congress). Washington, DC, U.S. Government Printing Office, 1967

Alexander CA: Physicians in the Department of Veterans Affairs. Arch Int Med 152:502–504, 1992

Association of American Medical Colleges: The Partnership: VA Hospitals and Graduate Medical Education. Washington, DC, Association of American Medical Colleges, 1990

Brown J: A veteran's vision. Federal Manager Quarterly 2:5–13, 1993

Charns MP, Tewksbury LS: Collaboration in Health Care: Implementing the Integrative Organization. San Francisco, Jossey Bass, 1993

Commission on the Future Structure of Veterans Health Care: Report of the Commission. Washington, DC, Department of Veterans Affairs, 1991

Department of Veterans Affairs: Biomedical Research. Washington, DC, Department of Veterans Affairs, 1993a

Department of Veterans Affairs: VA Mental Health Research. Washington, DC, Department of Veterans Affairs, 1993b

Errera P: From Yale professor to Washington bureaucrat: policy and medicine. VA Practitioner 81–93, 1988

Errera P: Psychiatry programs at VACO. VA Practitioner 41–50, 1992

Fisher ES, Welch HG: The future of the VA health care system. JAMA 273:651–655, 1995

Fontana A, Rosenheck R, et al. The long journey home: fifth program report on DVA's specialized PTSD programs. West Haven, CT, VAMC—Northeast Program Evaluation Centers, 1996 (182)

Frisman LK, Rosenheck R, Chapdelaine JD: Health care for homeless veterans: the ninth annual report. West Haven, CT, VAMC—Northeast Program Evaluation Center, 1996 (182).

Froelicher VF: How academic medicine and the VA are being influenced by changes in health-care delivery. Chest 110:239–242, 1996

General Accounting Office: Effectively implementing the Government Performance and Results Act (GADY/ggd-96-118). 1996a

General Accounting Office: VA health care: opportunities for service delivery efficiencies within existing resources (GAO/HEHS-96-121). 1996b

Gronvall JA: The VA's affiliation with academic medicine: an emergency postwar strategy becomes a permanent partnership. Acad Med 61–66, 1989

Hollingsworth JW, Bondy PK: The role of Veterans Affairs hospitals in the health care system. N Engl J Med 322:1851–1857, 1990

Iglehart JK: The Veterans Administration medical care system and the private sector. N Engl J Med 313:1552–1556, 1985

Iglehart JK: Reform of the Veterans Affairs health care system. N Engl J Med 335:1407–1411, 1996

Kizer KW: Vision for Change: A Plan to Restructure the Veterans Health Administration. Washington, DC, Department of Veterans Affairs, 1995

Kizer KW: Prescription for Change: The Guiding Principles and Strategic Objectives Underlying the Transformation of the Veterans Health Care System. Washington, DC, Department of Veterans Affairs, 1996a

Kizer KW: Transforming the Veterans health care system—the "new VA." JAMA 277:1069, 1996b

Magnuson PB: Ring the Night Bell. Boston, Little, Brown, 1960

Moos RH, Plette JD, Balsden KL: Health services for VA substance abuse patients: eight year trends in utilization. Palo Alto, CA, VA—Program Evaluation and Resource Center, 1996a

Moos RH, Humphreys K, Hamilton EG: Substance abuse treatment in the Department of Veterans Affairs: system structure, patients and treatment activities. Palo Alto, CA, VA—Program Evaluation and Resource Center, 1996b

National Center for Posttraumatic Stress Disorder: Sixth annual report FY 1995. White River Junction, VT, VA—National Center for Posttraumatic Stress Disorder, 1995

Petersdorf R: Report of the Residency Realignment Advisory Committee. Washington, DC, Department of Veterans Affairs, 1996

Rosenheck R: National Mental Health Program Performance monitoring system: FY 95 report for DVA. West Haven, CT, VA—Northeast Program Evaluation Center (182), 1996

Rosenheck R, Massari L: Wartime military service and utilization of VA health care services. Mil Med 158:223–228, 1993

Schafer J: Different drummers beckon as VA hospital system marches into the future. J Investig Med 44:179–189, 1996

Senate Veterans Affairs Committee: VA Mental Health Programs. Senate Hearing. Washington, DC, U.S. Government Printing Office, 1993, pp 103–314

Skocpol T: Protecting Soldiers and Mothers: The Beginnings of U.S. Social Policy. New York, WW Norton, 1992

Skocpol T: Boomerang: The Clinton Health Security Effort and the Turn Against Government in U.S. Politics. New York, WW Norton, 1996

Special Committee for Seriously Mentally Ill Veterans: Report to the undersecretary for health. Washington, DC, Department of Veterans Affairs, 1995

Special Committee for Seriously Mentally Ill Veterans: Report of the undersecretary to Congress. Washington, DC, Department of Veterans Affairs, 1997

CHAPTER 7

Summary of the Case Studies and Recommendations

Roger E. Meyer, M.D., and Christopher J. McLaughlin

This chapter summarizes some of the highlights of the case studies, as well as conclusions and recommendations drawn from preceding sections of this book. As described at the outset, the issues facing academic psychiatry departments are both generically similar to, and specifically different than, issues facing other clinical departments within the same academic health centers (AHCs). Managed behavioral health care is influencing the clinical income and educational environment of academic psychiatry in ways that are similar to the impact of managed health care on other clinical specialties. Clinical revenue per full-time equivalent (FTE) per hour is down in intensively managed care settings, and departments are being challenged to develop new models of clinical education that are compatible with the new health care environment. However, in many of the psychiatry departments that responded to the survey, professional fee billings account for a relatively minor (albeit significant) percentage of departmental income. Apart from professional fees for inpatient care in some departments in the 1980s, there has probably not been a time when "surplus" clinical income could provide significant support for the unfunded or underfunded costs of research and education in psychiatry. In many academic settings today, the structure, fees, and support services of the faculty practice plan (and the usual methodology for calculating bed charges) substantially handicap the psychiatry department as it tries to compete with the private sector. These difficulties have become more acutely burdensome in the context of managed behavioral health care, especially where psychiatry is being tithed for support services (e.g., appointment scheduling and managed care marketing) that fail to serve the needs of its practice.

It is curious that while most chairs tout the reconnection of their specialty to the rest of medicine, in many locations the potential role of psychiatry in organizing and overseeing all behavioral and psychosocial services throughout emerging academic health care systems is not being exploited. In ways that are probably unique among academic clinical departments, psychiatry in a number of AHCs is dependent on its relationship with the public sector to meet its educational responsibilities and to advance its research programs. Finally, psychiatry's emergence as a research-intensive clinical specialty over the past 15 years has substantially altered the criteria for academic excellence within the discipline.

At the outset of this study, we were pessimistic about the future of academic psychiatry. In truth, the glass is as full as it is empty. One cannot be pessimistic about an academic discipline with a rich variety of funded research opportunities and the promise of major new breakthroughs in neuroscience and genetics. At the same time, to quote a clinician colleague, "what is good for psychiatry may not be especially good for psychiatrists." If the clinical base of the specialty is eroded, what is the purpose of its clinical educational programs? The reality is that the clinical practice of psychiatry is changing. In the context of population-based integrated health–mental health care and a viable public sector, there are real opportunities for psychiatrists. Within academic settings, there is a need to grasp these changes and to advance the accountability of clinical practice for functional outcomes, quality of care, and sensitivity to costs. The case studies and the quotes of some of the successful department chairs reported in earlier chapters highlight some successful innovative strategies that have emerged and contrast with the problems highlighted in some of the cases. In the following sections we describe some general principles that the leaders of AHCs and of academic psychiatry might consider as they ponder the future.

Structure and Culture as Destiny

It should be axiomatic that the success of an academic psychiatry department is constrained by the sensitivity and responsiveness of the leadership and the relevance of the operational support structures within the parent AHC, as well as by the culture of the practice and the academic environment. The case example from Stanford is illustrative. Stanford's medical school has emphasized strong basic research programs since it moved to Palo Alto in the late 1950s. Commencing with the chairmanship of David Hamburg in the early 1960s, the psychiatry department has been firmly embedded within this tradition. For many years, the faculty appointments process within the university discouraged recruitment of clinician teachers. The Stanford University Hospital grew to depend on nearby practice groups and specialists for a substantial part of its clinical activity, and the medical school relied on many of these same resources for its clinical teaching. The faculty practice plan never really developed a true multispecialty group mentality or governance structure. The practice environment favored the development of some high-tech services, such as cardiac and other transplant surgery, while discouraging the clinical development of primary care, psychiatry, and interdisciplinary or interdepartmental centers of excellence (as in the care of patients with cancer).

Commencing in the mid-1980s under the deanship of David Korn and the presidency of Donald Kennedy, Stanford sought to recruit some clinical department heads who would expand the base of clinical activity and clinical research within the medical school. Efforts to expand the primary care base began in the early 1990s as a joint effort of Stanford University Hospital and the medical school. The recruitment of a new department head in psychiatry in the early 1990s, with an explicit mandate to expand the base of clinical activity and clinical research in the specialty, was consistent with these trends. In the context of this recruitment, the hospital opened new inpatient resources, and the university constructed a handsome new building for outpatient, partial hospital, and clinical research efforts. Unfortunately, these developments took place as managed care was beginning to impact substantially on the clinical environment in Northern California. In this context, the overall clinical income to the department could not cover the extremely high charges within a traditional faculty practice plan structure or the high allocated costs for the new facility. A substantial increase in industry-supported clinical research in psychiatry did not include indirect cost support for space or for the infrastructure of the university or department.

The installation of a new president at the university led to the departure of the dean and the hospital chief executive officer. The new leadership has since reemphasized Stanford's traditional commitment to high-tech tertiary and quaternary care and a lack of interest in primary care. Within this environment, psychiatry's recent successes in developing strong clinical programs, clinical education, and clinical research are not given significant weight. While the department has generated a substantial number of National Institutes of Health (NIH) and industry grants for its clinical research, it will need new resources to rebuild its basic science programs for the twenty-first century.

The case study highlights the ways in which the structure of the clinical practice environment and the culture underlying faculty development have served to constrain the possibilities for academic psychiatry. The lack of a connection to a significant public-sector program and a now problematic relationship with the local administration of the Veterans Administration (VA) medical center (which has recently been hostile to the traditional academic relationship with Stanford) serves to complete the picture. To the outside observer, the department of psychiatry under the leadership of its chair has been reasonably successful within the structure and culture of its AHC. In this environment, the department's vision of excellence in psychiatric clinical education, clinical research, and clinical practice may not be consistent with the direction of the medical center.

The University of Louisville School of Medicine's structure and culture provide an interesting contrast to Stanford. The university places no limits on physician income, and there is no centralized practice plan structure. There is a 3.45% dean's tax on individual net income from professional services, but accountability for oversight of each individual account rests at the departmental level. Each department is also able to tax the separate accounts for a departmental academic enhancement fund. Such an environment offers real autonomy to department heads within the practice environment, who are in a strong position to pick and choose areas of clinical emphasis. In this type of setting, tertiary clinical delivery has thrived, alongside traditional primary care and indigent care within outreach programs in Western Kentucky. There appears to be a pragmatic attitude toward the clinical departments within the school and among the principal nonprofit-affiliated hospitals. There are no major constraints on the recruitment of active clinicians and clinician teachers to the full-time faculty. The linkages between the medical school and its principal affiliated nonprofit hospitals were recently strengthened when the affiliation between the school and Humana Corporation (in the management of the university hospital) was terminated.

Psychiatry has been able to craft a vision linked to the public sector within this pragmatic environment, but it has not been able to bring a strong perspective on psychosocial and behavioral health services to the tertiary care programs. A new department head recruited in the early 1990s has elected to avoid the low discounted fee-for-service and capitation rates offered by managed behavioral health care and to link the clinical programs under his direction to the public sector. He has also strengthened clinical education for residents and medical students. The employment opportunities for psychiatrists in the area support a sense of optimism regarding the future stability of the residency program.

However, psychiatry has been constrained in its efforts to develop a clinical neuroscience program in this setting. In spite of 3 years of funding for a laboratory for a promising young research psychiatrist, the absence of proximal scientific colleagues has served to limit this research effort. There is no strong research tradition in the medical school and no basic neuroscience program. As much as the culture at Stanford supports the image of individual research laboratories supported and funded by investigator-initiated (R01) grants, this type of vision will face major obstacles at the University of Louisville.

The departments of psychiatry at the University of Maryland and the University of Colorado had histories of strong public sector–academic relationships prior to the arrival of new department heads in the mid-1980s. At the University of Colorado, the funding for public-sector programs was consistent with a tradition of indigent care within the academic health center. A separate budget for the Colorado Psychiatric Hospital comes to the university to support education, indigent care, and research in relationship to mental illness. While the chair of psychiatry reports to the dean of the medical school on academic issues, he also reports directly to the chancellor of the University of Colorado Health Sciences Center because of the distinct place of the Colorado Psychiatric Hospital within the health sciences center. This structure places the chair of psychiatry within the most senior leadership group at this AHC. It has also enabled the psychiatry department to negotiate case-based rates under managed care, because the chair is able to set bed charges and professional fees. Despite traditional deficiencies in support services to the department of psychiatry from the faculty practice plan (e.g., in managed behavioral health care marketing), the department has been able to craft a managed care–oriented service among its clinical programs.

The chair of psychiatry at the University of Colorado has also been able to amplify the department's role in the public sector through mutually beneficial contracts that staff the two state hospitals with faculty-appointed psychiatrists. Recently, the chair was asked to provide leadership in the state's efforts to privatize Medicaid and its behavioral health services. The structure of the public sector–academic relationship (and of psychiatric programs within the health sciences center at Colorado) has helped to advance the department's public-sector programs and managed care activities. The amplification of this structure, through the leadership skills of the chair, has brought psychiatry to a highly influential position within the AHC. At various times over the past decade, the head of psychiatry has also served as acting chancellor, acting vice chancellor, and acting chief executive officer of the university hospital, with other senior professors in the department also playing important roles within the institution.

Conversely, one is struck by the degree to which collaborative approaches to education in primary care and psychiatry have not been welcomed by primary care departments. At one level, this uncooperativeness probably is defined by the culture within the primary care departments. However, the psychiatry department has a small consultation-liaison service covering the VA and the university hospital, and only a half-time consultation-liaison psychiatrist working in the ambulatory care area. Despite psychiatry's prominent place within the health sciences center, the department is not involved to a significant degree in the oversight of psychosocial services and has not benefited from the managed care contracting efforts being charted by the head of the university hospital.

Finally, the broad range of research thriving within the department is consistent with a culture at the health sciences center that supports interdepartmental and interdisciplinary efforts. The vision of excellence and collegiality within the research environment also reflects the values of the chair and the associate chair for research. A strong budgetary situation, sustained by the public-sector relationship, has helped to foster new research initiatives and to cushion research programs caught between grant cycles. The department's high-quality mentoring of junior faculty should serve as a model to the field.

The case study from the University of Maryland serves as a useful echo to the University of Colorado on the importance of the public sector–academic relationship. At Maryland, this relationship is well understood and supported politically by the leadership of the University of Maryland–Baltimore campus, the hospital, and the medical school. The Maryland program has strengthened the quality of care throughout the public sector, while enabling the department to develop a very strong clinical and services research program within its educational mission. Before the arrival of the new department head in the mid-1980s, the department's identity had become diffused away from the campus of the AHC and into the geographically distributed public-sector program. The new chair embraced the broad commitment to the public sector but managed to anchor the identity of the department within the AHC environment. Yet within this setting, professional fee income is much less important to the department than public-sector contracts and research grants.

Like the University of Colorado, the department's efforts to cope with managed behavioral health care have been developed within a portion of its delivery system, as its bottom line has been protected by public-sector contracts. The linkage with the public sector has also been critical to the department in the development of its clinical research program in schizophrenia at the Maryland Psychiatric Research Center at Spring Grove State Hospital and in its neuroendocrine research programs at the VA medical center. The research environment on this campus has been very supportive of the department's clinical and services research programs.

Since 1984, the University of Maryland Hospital has been a 501(c)3 corporation, which has enabled it to function more effectively in the private sector than it had under state rules. The regulatory environment in Maryland has served to subsidize indigent care provided in the hospital (as in all general hospitals). The faculty practice plan is also a 501(c)3 corporation, but it has not evolved into a multispecialty group and many of its support services are not relevant to psychiatry. The hospital and practice plan have collaborated in the development of a health care program for university employees, and the department of family medicine has capitated contracts for 7,000 covered lives. The clinical leadership team at the medical center projects the development of a geographically distributed network of university-associated practices that will be brought together through a common contracting mechanism rather than through purchase of practices. The governing structure of this AHC provides the benefits of a state university without the usual state rules that discourage entrepreneurial activity in relationship to organized practice activity.

Recently the department of psychiatry has moved to align its clinical programs with those of the hospital, faculty practice plan, and department of family medicine. The division of alcohol and drug abuse (addictions) has placed consultants within the family practice ambulatory areas and in the employee assistance program for university employees. The head of this division has recently been named by the psychiatry chair to be head of a new division of behavioral health. This structural change was designed to offer a single point of accountability in the department to work with the clinical leadership of the medical center on managed care activities. The division's plans to develop an associated network of mental health clinicians conform well with the medical center's model of a network of associated community-based faculty across primary care disciplines.

The attitudes of the department chair and the new division director for managed care in psychiatry fit well with the cultural expectations of the evolving practice environment of the medical center. The traditional consultation-liaison service has been less effective in getting beyond traditional inpatient consultation psychiatry, and the changes being urged on psychiatry faculty by the chair and new division director are not being welcomed by advocates of a traditional view of psychiatric education, skills, and roles. At this juncture, the conflict of clinical and academic cultures is playing out within the department, rather than between the department and its medical center. The challenge to leadership in this circumstance will be to highlight the need for faculty attitudinal change in the context of emergent economic pressures and the inculcation of new practice patterns that will be responsive to the new health care environment.

The case study from Dartmouth describes its successful effort at engaging all psychiatry faculty to work within the changing health care delivery system. To some extent, the multispecialty group practice culture at Dartmouth-Hitchcock Medical Center could be said to facilitate this type of effort, but until recently it had not happened. Like the other case examples, the history of the department of psychiatry was largely shaped by its reporting relationship (structure) within the culture of the Dartmouth-Hitchcock Medical Center; the chair of psychiatry reports to the dean of Dartmouth Medical School.[1]

All other clinical departments are accountable for their budgets through the Lahey-Hitchcock Clinic. While the structure has enabled psychiatry to secure excellent public-sector contracts that might not have been possible in a traditional multispecialty practice environment, it has also made psychiatry "different." As a consequence, the department was not part of the clinic's strategic planning efforts for behavioral health services, nor was it involved in the Mary Hitchcock Memorial Hospital's behavioral health network with a group of affiliated community mental health centers. The department had its own linkage to the public sector through contracts with the New Hampshire State Hospital in Concord and a community mental health center in Manchester. As described, the disconnects were real and reflected the structural realities of the practice environment.

---

[1] Until recently, the chair of family and community medicine also had this reporting relationship, but now reports to the board of the Lahey-Hitchcock Clinic.

In the past 36 months, the chair and new faculty leadership have determined that there are two problems with the traditional clinical delivery system in the department: access and limited clinical capacity. Both served to make the department relatively less relevant to the pace of clinical practice within the medical center. Having identified structural and cultural impediments to its potential role within the larger medical center, the department's leadership decided to change the culture and structure of its own practice. The leaders in psychiatry at Dartmouth established a hierarchy of values for their delivery system: 1) ease of access to patients and referring physicians; 2) speed of assessment, diagnosis, treatment, or referral; and 3) a disease-management orientation focused on functional goals, costs of care, and patient satisfaction. They also incorporated a new model of residency education within the new clinical delivery system. The practice environment in the Lebanon, New Hampshire, division of the multispecialty Lahey-Hitchcock Clinic and the Mary Hitchcock Memorial Hospital was receptive to the innovative multidisciplinary diagnostic and longitudinal treatment teams.

The preliminary good news from the changes at Dartmouth suggest that a responsive clinical delivery system in psychiatry can shape psychosocial and behavioral health services within a practice environment that has a multispecialty group mentality (rather than the traditional federated or departmentally based structure of most faculty practice plans). Armed now with a new model of clinical service delivery at the AHC campus, the department is positioned to begin to work with a geographically distributed multispecialty practice group on the one hand and with the public sector on the other hand, as these two areas of activity cope with an increasing percentage of managed care. Finally, like the University of Colorado and the University of Maryland, the department at Dartmouth-Hitchcock Medical Center has benefited from a strong public sector–academic relationship that has helped to support its research efforts. In the case of Dartmouth, the public-sector relationship has helped to support a services research effort in relationship to chronic mental illness. The services research program is fully compatible with a strong tradition of services research at Dartmouth, especially in the department of medicine.

Cultural Change in Academic Psychiatry

The problems facing departments of psychiatry in many AHCs could serve as a case study in one of the texts by W. Edwards Deming (1993), who has highlighted the cultural and structural problems confronting a number of American industries and corporations in the context of changing markets and technology. His work has emphasized the need for systems to focus on continuous quality improvement through objective analysis of the structural and cultural impediments to effective change. The problems facing academic psychiatry are a microcosm of the problems facing AHCs that have been structured to maintain the culture of the status quo for as long as possible (Korn 1996).

If the parent medical center is gearing up for real change, departments of psychiatry need to position themselves to play an important role in the change process. If the changes in the institution are more apparent than real, the leadership of the department and of the medical center need to assess the structural problems that confront academic psychiatry in an effort to enable the department to meet its mission more effectively. Without question, the first lesson to be drawn from the case studies is that if there is a conflict between the culture of the psychiatry department and the parent medical center, it is easier to change the culture of the former than of the latter. Two recommendations are worthy of note.

Recommendation 1

If there is no centralized multispecialty faculty practice plan (which functions in the manner of a true group practice), there is a strong possibility that the allocated costs and the support structures are not functional for psychiatry and that the full potential of psychiatry in the oversight and direction of all psychosocial and behavioral health services is not being realized. Regardless of whether the practice plan functions as a multispecialty group, the leadership of the medical center and of the department should consider creating a separately budgeted and managed behavioral health product line structure that can develop case-based rates for managed care, accept capitation, support network develop-

ment, identify opportunities for joint ventures, develop contracts with
the public sector, provide direction and oversight for psychosocial services within the health care system of the AHC, and be held to standards
of clinical productivity and achievable financial targets. The clinical practice support system (i.e., managed care marketing, contracting, and
billings and collections) and costs should be relevant for psychiatric
practice. If the psychiatry department wishes to become involved in the
broad oversight of psychosocial and behavioral health services throughout the medical center and in a rapidly growing ambulatory and primary
care environment, it will need to rethink and restructure its traditional
approach to consultation-liaison psychiatry.

Recommendation 2

The optimal structure for a stable public sector–academic relationship
involves a predictable transfer of funds to the university for payment of
doctoral-level faculty within the program. The funding should bundle
support for the clinical, educational, and research components of the
effort. Programs identified as line items subject to an annual appropri-
ation are highly vulnerable to significant cuts or elimination. The public
sector–academic relationship is of such importance to the academic mission of many departments of psychiatry that it should engage the efforts
of the parent medical center or university in advocacy with state officials.

Managed Behavioral Health Care: Coping With Change

The six case studies offer six somewhat different approaches to managed
behavioral health care. As a freestanding psychiatric hospital, Sheppard-
Pratt has sought to transform itself into an integrated behavioral health
care delivery system capable of accepting capitated contracts, discounted
fee-for-service rates, employee assistance program activity, and benefits
management for employers. It has embraced public-sector patients and
merged its residency training program with the University of Maryland
to reduce the costs of education. It has adapted itself for its core mission

of clinical service and benefited from its ability to change or discard dysfunctional or irrelevant support services. No academic psychiatry department has this degree of latitude. Within academic psychiatry, chairs who are at least able to bring together all essential elements in contract negotiations with managed behavioral health care companies are in the best position to cope with the current and emerging clinical environment. Lacking this capability, the chair at Stanford negotiated with a local mental health group practice to market the specialized assessment and pharmacotherapy services of his department. The chairs at Colorado and the University of California–San Francisco (UCSF) are able to negotiate case-based rates for all aspects of their service delivery systems. The chair at UCSF is able to do it without the confounding burden of a faculty practice plan. The department at Northwestern has been able to reconfigure services in a profitable way in the context of a clinical practice environment that is closer to a multispecialty practice group.

Finally, as academic medical centers compete for managed health care business, some are learning that behavioral health services may have been carved out by prior agreement with a for-profit company that does not do business with their own academic departments of psychiatry. Conversely, some academic departments have developed preferred provider relationships or joint venture opportunities with specific managed behavioral health care companies. It is important to note that all managed behavioral health companies are not the same. According to a recent publication (Managed Behavioral Health Market Share in the United States 1996), the 4 largest companies together account for 54% of the market, the next 7 account for another 28.5% of the market, and the remaining 18 account for the rest. Although many of the initial heads of the companies had a clinical background, this preparation is currently less common. Ownership of many of the companies has changed over time—and will eventually impact on the direction of managed behavioral health care. As described in Chapter 2, Northwestern University Hospital owns one of the smaller behavioral health management companies, as does Sheppard-Pratt. In general, however, ownership of some of the larger companies varies from chains of for-profit hospitals to large health maintenance organizations (HMOs) to Wall Street entrepreneurs with no background in health care. The relatively rapid rate of turnover in management and ownership of these companies in the past few years makes it difficult to establish stable relationships (or joint venture partnerships) with them. On the other hand, as intense price competition in some health care markets has raised questions of quality of care, some managed behavioral health care companies may find their interests increasingly convergent with academic departments of psychiatry that have developed cost-effective and accountable delivery systems. There are two additional recommendations that may be drawn at this time.

Recommendation 3

The separation of managed behavioral health care from other managed care activities confronts AHCs in ways that can subvert integrated patient care. This separation constitutes a real threat to the clinical programs in academic psychiatry departments. Rather than being reactive, the times call for strategies that foster integration of patient care.

Recommendation 4

There is no single strategy to deal with change. Rather than change its corporate culture, General Motors invented the Saturn Corporation. Other companies in similar circumstances have attempted a total transformation of their workforce and practices. Still other companies have accepted a smaller niche market as the price for maintaining a valued cultural environment. The case examples describe a reinvention model (Maryland and Colorado), a model showing an attempt at total transformation (Sheppard-Pratt and Dartmouth), and a relatively status quo model (Louisville).

Leadership

Today, as some observers of AHCs decry their traditional departmental structure as an impediment to change (Kralewski et al. 1995), the case studies highlight the importance of departmental leadership in moving a faculty toward a new vision. Each of the chairs in the case studies presents an example of leadership in challenging times and settings. At Stanford, new leadership has highlighted the importance of clinical education in the residency training program and of clinical research among the faculty. It has brought pride in the quality of clinical service to a department in which clinical service had been considered relatively insignificant within the academic environment. At Louisville, new leadership has brought a focus on medical student and resident education, enabling the residency program to fill with United States medical school graduates, countering the current trend. Established leadership at Dartmouth brought in change agents to manage systemwide transformations. The latter process necessarily produced tension, but the leadership was sensitive to feedback from faculty and trainees. Colorado and Maryland were refurbished, helping to heal the problems of morale and faculty conflict to restore a vision of public sector–academic collaboration and research excellence. Finally, leadership at Sheppard-Pratt has transformed a traditional psychiatric hospital for the relatively affluent into a behavioral health system that serves the broader community.

In a time of declining resources, leadership is challenged throughout academic institutions to consider the interests of the larger enterprise. Deans and vice presidents of AHCs are urged by university presidents to protect the financial well-being of the parent universities, which have derived significant financial support for their administrative, research, and educational infrastructure from once-profitable academic medical centers over the past four decades. As the latter are forced to downsize and reduce costs to meet budgets, tensions can develop between the medical center and its university, as well as among the legitimate interests of the medical school, other health science schools, the hospital, the practice plan, and individual departments. At medical schools and hospitals that once invested resources in recruiting clinical and research superstars to departmental leadership positions, there is a growing appreciation of leaders who are team players rather than outstanding soloists. Leadership is being clearly challenged at every level, and the intrinsic tensions partially account for the recent high turnover of medical school deans.

In a competitive corporate world, employees can be mobilized by setting performance standards. Employees are expected to perform as

they are told. Management of faculty performance is not so straightfor-
ward.[2] It requires a careful balance of team building, responsible advocacy for faculty interests by departmental and institutional leaders, and
demonstrated commitment to the goals of the institution by these same
individuals. The balance was well articulated by the chair at Colorado,
who demonstrated the art of team building in his advocacy for (and
mentorship of) younger faculty that had become part of the departmental culture. By withholding substantial objection to the problems
presented to his department's clinical programs by the hospital's managed care marketing strategies, or the costs of inappropriate services
charged by the practice plan, he reinforced his identity as a team player.
He had previously established his credentials in this regard by his voluntary service in a variety of acting administrative positions in the institution. As a recognized team player, he could be a more effective
advocate for the department's core interest in maintaining the administrative autonomy of the Colorado Psychiatric Hospital.

   While the balance of emphasis at Colorado is consistent with its
structure, these three dimensions (team building, departmental advocacy, and institutional team player) are important to all department
heads. Deans, vice presidents, and hospital chief executive officers also
face the same challenges. Team building requires effective communication throughout the institution, but the traditional forums (faculty senate, departmental meetings, and meetings of department heads with
hospital chief executive officers and deans) do not serve this function to
an adequate degree. Communication is necessarily a two-way process in
which institutional leaders communicate goals and objectives and are
responsive to feedback from the faculty on the ways in which change is
shifting their roles.

   Communication is also critical in establishing a credible case for
fairness and equity within the system. This sense of fairness is essential
during a time when faculty will be expected to work harder for uncertain rewards. Administration needs to demonstrate its own accountability in the performance of support services and in its willingness to
sacrifice. In a time of crisis, faculty and staff need to feel that they are
appreciated. With tenure providing job security for the most senior

---

[2] Indeed, it has been likened to "herding cats."

faculty, departmental and institutional leaders are challenged to develop balanced expectations from all faculty, lest excessive burdens fall on junior faculty whose academic careers would be prematurely shortened in inequitable systems.

Recommendation 5

Leadership of an academic psychiatry department today requires a vision that is aware of the dangers, anticipates the possibilities, motivates the faculty, and engages the support of the principal stakeholders (medical school, hospital, and public-sector leadership) in an effort that requires constant attention without micromanagement. It requires realistic levels of optimism and a will to prevail despite occasional setbacks. The successful leader develops a vision compatible with the values of the time and of the area of practice. Departmental leadership must be sensitive to the needs of the entire institution by advocating for departmental goals within the context of institutional strategies.

Education

Nearly all of the respondent departments of psychiatry, and all of the case study departments, are involved in the education of medical students, nonpsychiatric physicians,[3] psychiatric residents and advanced clinical and research fellows, and other mental health professionals. Louisville and Colorado have been very successful at reaching medical students and interesting a significant number in psychiatry. This connection has been an important factor in enabling these departments to attract a cadre of excellent United States medical school graduates to their residency programs (starting with their own students). At Colorado, a member of the psychiatry faculty has played a major role in curriculum reform and problem-based learning and recently received the Teacher of the Year Award for his teaching in the second-year curriculum. At

---

[3] Sheppard-Pratt is not involved in the education of nonpsychiatric physicians. It offers some education of medical students and is merging its GME programs with the University of Maryland.

Maryland, the chair of the committee overseeing problem-based learning is also a psychiatrist and a past Teacher of the Year Award recipient. Indeed, the introduction of a new curriculum founded on problem-based learning should be an optimal vehicle for introducing biopsychosocial concepts into medicine. At Louisville, the introduction of a longitudinal primary care sequence is seen by the department as an excellent vehicle to extend the teaching of psychiatry into other areas of ambulatory practice, a view supported by the chair of family medicine.

The psychiatry clerkship will continue to serve as the decision-making point for many students who might be considering careers in psychiatry. If the morale of key psychiatric educators is low, in the context of changes in patterns of practice and reimbursement, one can expect a decline in the percentage of graduates choosing the specialty. In the case studies, good faculty morale was related to an optimistic view of the department and the faculty members' own views of their present and future value as researchers, educators, and clinicians. Faculty who resented managed behavioral health care and identified strongly with the traditions of long-term psychotherapy in psychiatric education and practice felt pessimistic about the field's present directions.

In some ways, these faculty attitudes represent the most important challenge facing the leaders of academic psychiatry, lest the pessimism of these educators become a self-fulfilling prophecy. To prevent the recent decline of interest in psychiatry among United States medical school graduates from becoming a continuing downward spiral, students will have to be convinced of the scientific, clinical, and economic possibilities within the field, the opportunities for public service, and the quality of mentoring that they experience during the preclinical and clinical years. At places like Stanford and Colorado, the broad array of research opportunities and postresidency research fellowships may continue to attract medical school graduates interested in full-time academic careers. At places like Louisville, a strong mentoring program for its own medical students may encourage them to remain as residents.

However, the real challenge facing the field for the foreseeable future will be whether it is possible to embrace long-term psychotherapy as the gold standard of psychiatric practice in residency training programs when this treatment modality is not being covered by managed behavioral health companies (and is being offered by lower-cost mental health service providers). In their survey responses and in the case studies, the vast majority of chairs acknowledge the problem; but among the case study departments, only Dartmouth had successfully transformed itself to reflect a new practice identity within the training program. The "Firm Model" adopted by this program was also projected for the future by 10% of the survey respondents.

As described at the conclusion of Chapter 3, the real challenge to academic psychiatry, working in conjunction with the leaders of the managed behavioral health industry, will be to develop a credible intellectual foundation for population-based mental health care that will inform clinical practice. At its best, this effort will include meaningful roles and skills for *each* of the mental health disciplines within the interdisciplinary team construct. It will serve to amplify the roles of these professionals in the general health care system and offer realistic cost- and quality-sensitive models of patient care that are aimed at improving the functional capacities of patients with chronic and severe mental and addictive disorders. For psychiatry at this stage in its history, the practice model must be founded on a knowledge- and skill-based professionalism capable of advancing in the future in response to scientific understanding.

Regrettably, the past offers little reason to be hopeful about the future. Despite the 40 years psychopharmacology has existed, biological, psychodynamic, and social/community psychiatry have been taught to residents and medical students as discrete silos of knowledge. It was somehow expected that an integrated vision of patient care would emerge within each trainee. Indeed, patients and referring physicians could expect quite different treatment recommendations depending on the training program and the age of the psychiatrist. Leon Eisenberg (1986) has decried the shift from a "brainless psychiatry" to a "mindless psychiatry." Educators will be challenged to maintain a focus on the doctor-patient relationship and the importance of life history in shaping an understanding of the patient in his or her environment. Healing and recovery of function take place in a biopsychosocial context that must be learned if it is to be practiced. Whatever the future of managed behavioral health care, one hopes that it will leave psychiatry with a legacy of accountability for its educational and clinical results.

While the transformation of the content of residency training and the associated transformation of faculty attitudes toward new practice paradigms constitute the most critical challenges facing residency educators, departments also need to consider the impact of some less-qualified residents on the attitudes of medical students toward psychiatry. Should departments consider the advantages of recruiting a smaller number of higher quality residents to their training programs? Maryland/Sheppard-Pratt, Dartmouth, and Colorado have begun to seriously downsize their residency training programs. Maryland and Sheppard-Pratt have merged their training programs, thereby reducing the number of graduates and using the diminished teaching time of clinically active faculty more efficiently. Colorado has downsized its program within the context of the traditional public-sector programs at the Colorado Psychiatric Hospital. It will be challenged to modify these programs as they come under managed Medicaid behavioral health care carveouts.

Among the departments responding to the survey, plans for downsizing of residency programs seemed more modest. The leaders of the field need to consider workforce needs broadly, including the skills, roles, and need for psychiatrists, other mental health professionals, and primary care physicians with additional training in the treatment of mentally ill and addicted patients. At this juncture, there is no consensus on these issues (Eisenberg 1995; Guze 1992; Lieberman and Rush 1996).

Just as the 1980s were marked by an increase in residency positions in psychiatry, the 1990s have been characterized by the proliferation of postresidency fellowships across an array of newly accredited subspecialties (e.g., geriatric, addiction, forensic, and consultation-liaison psychiatry), as well as a growing interest in joint residency training programs leading to dual or triple board eligibility (e.g., psychiatry/neurology, psychiatry/family medicine, psychiatry/internal medicine, and adult and child psychiatry/pediatrics). Although the joint board programs have a certain intrinsic appeal relative to advancing the clinical neuroscience skills of psychiatrists who are joint board eligible in neurology (and of the primary care skills of psychiatrists who are joint board eligible in a primary care discipline), it remains to be seen whether these graduates identify themselves as practicing psychiatrists or as practitioners in their other specialty. If the latter manifests, it is not clear whether their education could have been advanced more effectively by incorporating more psychiatric teaching in the general neurology (or primary care) training program. Regrettably, it is too soon to judge the outcome of these dual board eligible programs based on the case study or survey materials.

The advanced clinical fellowship and the dual (or triple) board programs depend on hospital-based or other local resources for funding at a time when stipend support beyond the period required for single board eligibility (apart from geriatrics) is unlikely. The growth of subspecialty interest among psychiatric educators comes at a time when managed behavioral health care is emphasizing the skills of psychiatrists who can serve the broadest array of patients with mental and addictive disorders (i.e., generalists). The case study departments, in aggregate, reflect the trend toward subspecialization. Advanced clinical fellowship training at Maryland spans all of the subspecialty areas. The other case study departments offer advanced clinical fellowships in areas of perceived clinical expertise. There is no objective evidence that the identified subspecialties have had a significant impact on medical student interest in the field, at a time when medical students are being encouraged to avoid subspecialty training in other areas of medicine. Moreover, it is possible that clinical training experiences relevant to the new adult psychiatry subspecialties could be offered within reformatted general residency programs. In contrast to the advanced clinical fellowship programs, the advanced research fellowship programs in the more research-intensive departments (e.g., Stanford and Colorado) appear to be thriving. Support for these stipends usually comes from NIH-funded institutional training grants for research training.

Finally, while some departments are also known for their efforts in the continuing education of clinicians in practice, this dimension of the educational mission was not emphasized in any of the case studies or in the survey materials. Yet it is also clear from a managed care perspective that the continuing education of the existing workforce (including existing faculty) is a high priority. Of the case studies, only Dartmouth set out to clinically retool its faculty in a broad and systematic way (a component of continuing medical education [CME]). As departments begin to reconsider the size of their graduate medical education (GME) initiatives, they may be encouraged to undertake new CME initiatives— perhaps in conjunction with managed behavioral health care companies.

The broad educational responsibilities of academic psychiatry departments were affirmed in the case studies and survey materials. A number of possible recommendations stand out.

Recommendation 6

Problem-based learning and curriculum reform represent important opportunities for academic psychiatry departments to provide leadership on biopsychosocial and population-based aspects of the undergraduate curriculum. While several of the case study departments offer excellent examples of such leadership, there is cause for concern that the costs for these educational initiatives is buried within departmental budgets that will be strained under the financial impact of managed behavioral health care. Medical school administrators and clinical department heads need to identify the educational costs of faculty time in the core disciplines (including psychiatry) and develop strategies to meet some of these costs.

Recommendation 7

While most of the case study departments were not involved in educational consortia or collaborative telemedicine initiatives in their undergraduate, graduate, or GME programs, academic psychiatry departments should begin to develop more cost-effective collaborative models in their educational programs. The child development program in the Denver area is an example of the possibilities for child psychiatry education within a consortium model.

Recommendation 8

The problems confronting GME in psychiatry are broadly based and include overcapacity in residency slots, lack of consensus on changing residency curricula to address the relevant clinical skills and roles of psychiatrists in the context of managed behavioral health care, and low morale among faculty with traditional views of psychiatric education and practice. Departments will need to address these GME issues across the board.

Recommendation 9

The usefulness of joint board eligible programs and of subspecialty clinical fellowships need to be objectively evaluated before too many unfilled residency slots are converted into fellowship or dual residency programs.

Recommendation 10

CME represents an opportunity understood by some of the more enlightened leaders of managed behavioral health care companies. Their interest and financial resources need to be aligned more closely with the educational capacities of academic psychiatry departments.

Research

Chapter 4 highlighted the extraordinary growth of psychiatry as a research-intensive clinical discipline. The case studies serve to amplify some of the survey data, as well as the data from NIH on the research standing of departments of psychiatry and their parent medical schools. None of the case study departments overachieved or underachieved relative to the standing of their medical school. Stanford and Colorado were in the top quartile of NIH support among psychiatry departments, Maryland was just below the top quartile, Dartmouth was in the second quartile, and Louisville was in the lower half. None of the five departments has access to a positron-emission tomography (PET) scanner at their medical centers, although Maryland enjoys access through a nearby facility. Among the 45 departments that responded to the survey question on research resources, more than one-third of the departments in the top quartile did not have access to a PET scanner and 55% did not have access to a research single photon emission computed tomography (SPECT) scanner. At this stage, access to certain specific technologies does not delimit research productivity.

However, the future of basic psychiatric research will likely require institutional resources that are relevant to a number of areas of brain science as it relates to clinical medicine. As institutions look to limited funding to invest in new research resources, they will be obliged to

invest in technologies that can serve the interests of a number of
research-intensive departments. As the second-most-research-intensive
department in many medical schools, the psychiatry department needs
to be involved in this type of planning effort. As research in psychiatry
necessarily becomes more molecular, the critical priority for the field
will be the education of a new generation of clinically and scientifically
sophisticated investigators who are capable of applying the methods of
molecular biology to the problems of mental illness. These young investigators will also need to be able to secure the type of time available
to young research faculty in internal medicine if they are to advance
their science.

Public-sector support for research has been critical to the success
of the psychiatry departments at Colorado and Maryland, as to half of
the departments in the top 10 among NIH grant support and a number
of other departments in the top or second quartile. Dartmouth's highly
regarded services research program is partially supported by the public
sector. Public-sector support, the vision of the chair and the excellence
of the faculty, the culture and resources of the academic medical center
with respect to research, and the potential for developing strong research programs in special niche areas, such as addictions or AIDS, define
and delimit the research possibilities. Adequate resources and a departmental culture that can support the research career development of
younger faculty is critical to the long-term strength of the research
enterprise. The case study from Colorado, and the quote from the chair
at Pittsburgh (see Chapter 4), highlight the rich possibilities when these
elements are aligned with a research focus that spans many years. The
following recommendations highlight a part of the challenge.

Recommendation 11

Although strategic planning for research will not provide the specific
ideas or breakthroughs to generate new research grants, it will be increasingly critical for AHCs and departments that wish to remain research intensive. Planning is important in defining the essential infrastructure for research. Depending on their resources, psychiatry
departments may play an important (or collaborative) role in planning
for a number of potential areas of emphasis within an AHC, including

services research, clinical trials and investigation, human genetics, brain imaging, behavioral and psychosocial research, and a number of research areas within the broad interdisciplinary field of neuroscience.

Recommendation 12

Given limited resources, departments of psychiatry should explore intra- and interuniversity collaborations in research. They should fully explore possible public-sector (including VA) support for research on mental and addictive disorders.

Recommendation 13

Priority should be given to faculty research career development in research-intensive departments.

Recommendation 14

Niche research areas represent targets of opportunity for departments striving to become more research intensive. Innovative funding opportunities (foundations and charitable contributions) represent important new sources of support for psychiatric research.

Psychiatry and Primary Care

The case studies from Colorado, Dartmouth, Louisville, Maryland, and Stanford highlight the challenges that primary care and psychiatry departments face if they are to develop quality integrated service delivery programs for patients with mental and other medical disorders. The heads of the departments of family medicine at Louisville and Maryland welcomed input from psychiatry in the primary care practice sites. Family practice residents spend 1 month on psychiatry at Louisville, and a family practice resident is doing a substance abuse clinical fellowship at Maryland. At Dartmouth, the recent changes in ambulatory service consultations have had a dramatic impact on the perception of the psychiatry department's responsiveness. In all of these settings, the challenge will be to keep the momentum moving by assuring quick access by referring physicians and patients to mental health consultation and follow-through care. Dartmouth's recent reorganization has served to address both of these issues.

At the other end of the spectrum, primary care clinicians at Stanford feel like relative orphans. They tend to see psychiatry as another specialty service—and would welcome more input than the services of a senior resident. At Colorado, the primary care departments appear to respect their senior colleagues in psychiatry, even as they do not feel they need them to teach their residents in the ambulatory practice. The consultation-liaison services at Colorado and Stanford appear to be more traditionally focused on inpatient services, although a recent graduate has developed a half-time consultation practice in primary care at Colorado.

The survey data from the psychiatry chairs and from the primary care program heads in the case study departments suggest that there is a relatively high degree of consensus that primary care physicians should be able to diagnose and treat major depression and anxiety disorders. The primary care program heads were even more confident that their graduates could recognize and treat all psychiatric disorders except acute psychosis (including mania). Surprisingly, the literature does not support much optimism about the ability of primary care physicians to recognize or treat depression (or other psychiatric disorders), without substantial efforts to change the primary care practice environment (see Chapter 5). The literature also does not support the present ability of psychiatrists to offer primary care services to the chronically and severely mentally ill, although there is recognition that these services are vital to these patients. While the literature would suggest some potential directions for improvement, the case studies do not give a clear indication of how high-quality, well-integrated mental health and primary care services can be rendered under fee-for-service or carveout (or "carve-in") arrangements.

Recommendation 15

Because primary care and psychiatry departments do not have the resources to develop high-quality, well-integrated mental health and primary care services on their own, these efforts should be developed as part of the strategic clinical plans of AHCs. The resulting programs should be able to serve patients from fee-for-service, as well as carved-out, carved-in, and other managed care arrangements. Optimally, the resulting ambulatory care sites should be able to serve as training venues for primary care physicians, other primary care clinicians, psychiatrists, and other mental health professionals.

The Department of Veterans Affairs

The five case study departments reflect some of the changes going on in the Department of Veterans Affairs. A number of the strong clinical research programs in psychiatry at Stanford were based at the Palo Alto Veterans Affairs Hospital. In the past few years, pressure from a new director to apparently downplay the academic linkage has served to generate conflict between psychiatry faculty and the administration of the hospital. The problems have posed a threat to the ongoing viability of a schizophrenia research center supported by the National Institute of Mental Health (NIMH), as well as other major programs.

At Maryland, the leadership of the Veterans Integrated Service Network (VISN) has shut down the specialized units devoted to posttraumatic stress disorder (PTSD) and addictions, compromising funded research programs on these disorders. Similar problems have surfaced in other locations (e.g., the Manhattan VA Hospital). In contrast, the new chief of psychiatry at the Denver VA Hospital was very optimistic about the future opportunities for academic psychiatry at his facility. This optimism was also reflected in visits to Louisville and to White River Junction (a Dartmouth affiliate). As in the past, the Department of Veterans Affairs offers the appearance of a bureaucratic monolith, but local differences in administration account for different relationships between local VA hospitals and medical schools. The real prospects for the future must ultimately depend on decisions in the Congress and the support of veterans' services organizations.

In Chapter 6, Dr. Thomas Horvath, the Director of Mental Health Services in the VA, writes optimistically about the possibilities. Indeed, the new VISN structure has made it possible to have integrated planning for all mental health disciplines under unified leadership. While some have based the new VISN structure on a staff model HMO (with its emphasis on primary care and health promotion) (Kizer 1996), the real challenge to the VISN directors will be to convert a specialist-intensive workforce into a model disease-management system that can teach the private sector how to deliver high-quality, cost-efficient care to patients with chronic illnesses. Since the most prevalent disorders in the VA system are cared for by psychiatrists, these models should have great relevance to the field of psychiatry.

Recommendation 16

In many AHCs academic psychiatry departments have a symbiotic relationship with the local Department of Veterans Affairs hospital. In the short term, political efforts at the local and national level (in conjunction with veterans' services organizations) will be needed to assure veterans access to high-quality care in the context of a strong VA-academic linkage. Recent threatened closures of clinical units that link patient care and research on schizophrenia, addictive disorders, PTSD, and other conditions represent a major threat to patient care and research on these disorders.

Summary

Because it is more firmly a part of academic medicine than ever before, psychiatry is like one more passenger on a ship in a storm-tossed sea. As the leaders of AHCs attempt to develop sound approaches to the future, they are trying to eliminate unnecessary and unproductive tasks. However, because the costs of the academic mission have never been well documented, risky strategies could place the enterprise at risk. As an observer of a number of AHCs over the past 4 years, the senior author has developed some impressions and biases that may be both instructive and controversial. Whether or not the recommendations of the Pew Commission (1995) are followed, it is likely that a number of medical schools and teaching hospitals could close in the next 5 to 10 years—especially if the medical student applicant pool declines precipitously as undergraduates appreciate the economic and practice impact of managed care on the profession. If (or when) this decline occurs, the impact will probably first be felt among some private schools with the highest tuition rates and at some of the smaller campuses of publicly funded medical schools in the Midwest (if these states choose to consolidate their medical education programs to a smaller number of sites in order to gain greater savings).

More optimistically, some AHCs have managed to develop excellent strategies for the future. These strategies have been easier to implement in settings where there is a corporate linkage between the medical school or unified practice plan and the principal teaching hospital. This situation is further optimized by a reporting structure that links the profitability of the clinical enterprise to the academic mission. The hospital chief executive officer at Colorado put it well when he described the purpose of his "business" as the advancement of the academic mission of the AHC. At Colorado, the hospital is governed by a board of trustees chaired by the chancellor for health affairs, who can serve as a transducer between the corporate or clinical functions of the enterprise and the academic mission. The University of Maryland–Baltimore offers an analogous model. It seems Stanford currently lacks such a transducer (Andreopoulos 1997). There is also no one serving this function at Dartmouth, although the Hitchcock Clinic and the hospital have a long tradition of support for the medical school. In general, AHCs in which the principal teaching hospital has a separate governing structure from the medical school (which is governed by the university board) appear to be having a more difficult time in the new environment.

Some institutions appear to be confusing strategy and tactics. The simple sale of the principal teaching hospital to a for-profit hospital chain may serve as a short-term tactic designed to gather funds for the university or the AHC. In this scenario the hospital is being treated as a commodity and not as a core part of the academic enterprise. The strategic goals of the purchaser may be quite different from those of the AHC—acquiring the name and reputation of the latter to advance the credibility and profitability of the purchaser (or lessee) in a number of health care markets. The different objectives may also be reflected in significant differences in culture and values. Creighton University had to repurchase 20% ownership of the teaching hospital that it once owned in order to assure that the educational mission would continue under new for-profit ownership. It is not clear that the leadership of AHCs that have sold (or announced their intention to lease or sell) their teaching hospital actually visited Creighton or the University of Louisville to discuss the latter institution's relatively long experience with the management of its principal teaching hospital by Humana. As described by the vice president at Louisville, the promise of 20% of the annual profits never really materialized in the context of the management fees. In contrast, the present linkage of the medical school and hospital complex to a holding company developed by a partnership of the two other (nonprofit) affiliates on the same campus has brought strategic and substantial financial benefits to the school. It is certainly possible for nonprofit organizations to develop joint ventures with for-profit companies, but the venture needs to be seen in the context of a long-term strategy and not merely as a tactic to address a projected or short-term problem with the bottom line.

Downsizing by itself is also not a strategy. Downsizing of a university hospital that remains isolated in its principal market may actually do harm in the long term. However, downsizing in the context of a regional strategy that looks to a larger share of the market through joint ventures and other approaches can be quite helpful. As demonstrated by the University of Colorado (and in the plans being developed at Maryland), it may not be necessary to purchase primary care practices if one can develop a broad geographic network of facilities that can capture managed care contracts. The strategies at these two AHCs benefited from state affiliation, but it is possible that similar strategies could be crafted by private AHCs that have a unique cachet in their health care environment. As another option, the University of Pennsylvania has developed a regional strategy built around the purchase of geographically distributed primary care practices (Inglehart 1995).

Ultimately, AHCs need to develop budget-driven strategies that examine the real costs of their mission. Through a variety of strategies over the past 20 years, they have managed to prosper in spite of multiple government efforts at cost containment. Through Democratic and Republican administrations, the federal government found ways to help AHCs to meet their mission of education, research, and specialized patient care. Over time, academic medicine grew dependent on clinical income to help fund the other parts of its mission. With the growing corporatization of health care (including Medicaid and Medicare), the burden for holding the line on health care costs has fallen to corporate America, which likely cares more about its costs in a global economy than it does about the beneficence of new scientific knowledge and medical education. This attitude represents a major change in the health care environment for AHCs, which will have a hard sell linking higher patient care costs to unspecified costs of teaching and research. Academic psychiatry shares the responsibility with its counterparts in other academic departments to develop cost-efficient models of undergraduate medical education, to develop broad-based collaborations to support research, to practice medicine in cost-sensitive and outcome-accountable ways, and to educate the present workforce and appropriate numbers of future clinicians to follow these models of clinical practice.

References

Andreopoulos S: Sounding board: the folly of teaching hospital mergers. N Engl J Med 336:61–64, 1997

Deming WE: The New Economics: For Industry, Government, Education. Cambridge, MA, Massachusetts Institute of Technology, 1993

Eisenberg L: Mindlessness and brainlessness in psychiatry. Br J Psychiatry 148:497–508, 1986

Eisenberg L: The social construction of the human brain. Am J Psychiatry 152:1563–1575, 1995

Guze SB: Why Psychiatry Is a Branch of Medicine. New York, Oxford University Press, 1992.

Inglehart J: Academic medical center enters the market: the case of Philadelphia. N Engl J Med 333:1019–1023, 1995

Kizer K: Prescription for change: the guiding principles and strategic objectives underlying the transformation of the veterans healthcare system.1996

Korn D: Reengineering academic health centers: reengineering academic values? Acad Med 71:1033–1043, 1996

Lieberman JA, Rush AJ: Redefining the role of psychiatry in medicine. Am J Psychiatry 153:1388–1397, 1996

Managed Behavioral Health Market Share in the United States, 1996: Open Minds. Gettysburg, PA, 1996

Pew Health Professions Commission: Critical Challenges: Revitalizing the Health Professions for the Twenty-First Century. Pew Health Professions Commission, 1995

The Department of Psychiatry at the University of Colorado Health Sciences Center

Roger E. Meyer, M.D.

I visited the department of psychiatry at the University of Colorado Health Sciences Center on June 13–14, 1996. Within the health sciences center, I met with Dean Richard Krugman, M.D.; Mr. Dennis Brimhall, the president of the university hospital; and Mrs. Lilly Marks, the director of the faculty practice plan. In the department of psychiatry, I met with Dr. James Shore (chair), Dr. Robert House (director of the psychiatry residency training program and chief of the consultation-liaison service), Ms. Audrey County (administrator of the Colorado psychiatric hospital and of the department of psychiatry), Dr. Steven Dubovsky (vice chair for clinical affairs in the department of psychiatry and the Colorado Psychiatric Hospital), Dr. Robert Freedman (vice chair and director for research in the department of psychiatry), Dr. Martin Reite (chief of psychiatry at the Denver Veterans Administration Medical Center), and Dr. Marshall Thomas, (director of psychiatric acute care, managed care, and inpatient services at the Colorado Psychiatric Hospital).

Dr. Larry Green (chair, department of family medicine) provided

me with the perspective of a primary care department. Dr. Martin
Dubin (chief executive officer of PRO Behavioral Health Corporation)
offered the views of managed behavioral health, and Dr. Thomas Barrett
offered the perspective of the public mental health sector in Colorado.
In addition to those already mentioned, I had the opportunity to meet
with members of the executive committee of the department of psychiatry in a group meeting.

General Environment

The University of Colorado School of Medicine is the only medical
school in the state and functions as one of five health science schools on
the university's health sciences campus at Denver. The chancellor of the
University of Colorado health sciences center, Dr. Vincent Fulginiti,
reports to the president of the university and an elected board of regents.
Prior to 1991, there had been nine deans in the previous 12 years in
the school of medicine. The clinical programs were hampered by an
inadequate hospital physical plant. In the past five years, the school of
medicine and the hospital have made tremendous progress in developing
a strong leadership team, privatizing the hospital to make it administra-
tively and financially more effective, and strengthening the undergraduate medical education programs. The school of pharmacy has been
relocated from Boulder to a new building on the health sciences campus,
and a new hospital building with 300 staffed beds has been added. The
pediatric services have been consolidated at the Denver Children's Hospital.

A new ambulatory care building is being developed under the joint
sponsorship of the hospital and the faculty practice plan, and a handsome
new medical education center has recently been proposed. The director
of the hospital, Mr. Dennis Brimhall, serves as the "point person" in the
development of a new statewide network of providers: Health Care
Colorado. As described by Mr. Brimhall, the university hospital and
medical school are involved in the development of a virtual network,
which includes a core of facilities in the city of Denver and a developing
group of affiliations throughout the state. Within Denver, the core includes the Denver General Hospital and the Denver Health and Hospitals

Corporation, the National Jewish Hospital, University Physicians, Inc. (the faculty practice plan), the university hospital, Denver Children's Hospital, and the Colorado Psychiatric Hospital. The Colorado Psychiatric Hospital is one of the equity owners of Health Care Colorado. Each of the equity owners in the state has contributed $50,000 toward the initial organizational effort.

The Denver metropolitan area is described by the University Health-System Consortium (UHC) as one of the most intensively managed care environments in the country. Columbia HCA has become a major competitor to the university hospital through the acquisition of a number of highly regarded previously nonprofit hospitals in the city. A second major provider network consists of hospitals associated with the Catholic archdiocese in the state. The university hopes that Health Care Colorado, the system that it is nurturing, will become the third major provider network. Through its participation in the virtual network, the university hopes to be part of a managed care system that could be responsible for 300,000 to 350,000 covered lives in the next 12 to 18 months. It is already involved in providing capitated health care coverage to employees of the University of Colorado (15,000 members) and hopes to be selected as part of a consortium (Tri West) that is competing for a CHAMPUS contract. This move would bring in an additional 130,000 covered lives. The university is also hoping to be selected, along with its Denver-based and statewide partners, for the managed Medicaid program in Colorado (Colorado Access). Finally, there is additional hope that the university will be able to compete for the managed care business of all employees of colleges and universities in the state and state employees. The proposed efforts at securing managed Medicaid activity, as well as higher education and state employees, are consistent with a strong historical commitment to indigent care and the health of the citizens of Colorado (the core mission of the school of medicine, university hospital, and the Colorado Psychiatric Hospital).

The faculty practice plan is governed by a board of directors that consists of the department chairs of the major clinical departments on a nonrotational basis and department chairs of smaller departments on a rotational basis. The dean serves as the chair of the faculty practice plan organization. There is a separate medical director. The faculty practice plan (University Physicians, Inc.) charges a series of fees associated with different types of departmental income. These fees include an academic enhancement fund (AEF) assessment of 10% of income from patient care, clinical contract dollars received from the university hospital for professional services rendered to medically indigent patients, medical legal income, and clinical service contracts where the physician performs clinical services in outside entities and is reimbursed. There is no AEF assessment on contract dollars related to outside administrative service by a physician, contract dollars provided to a department for a portion of a physician's salary from outside entities, and interest income earned on investments.

A sliding scale of administrative assessments for the operation of the practice plan ranges from 9% of income received for patient care services to 3% on clinical contract dollars received from the university hospital for indigent care, medical legal income, and clinical services contracts. There is also a 3% administrative assessment on investment income and a 1% assessment on contract dollars received from outside entities in relationship to the performance of administrative services by a full-time faculty member. Where departments plan to use any of the mentioned sources of income to supplement faculty salaries, there is a 22% charge for fringe benefits.

University Physicians, Inc., provides central administrative services, including billing and collections and managed care contracting for all departments. Psychiatry does not participate in the centralized appointments system, and only 35% of outpatient billings in psychiatry are directly processed by University Physicians, Inc. The latter also does not provide managed care marketing for psychiatry, which handles this task on its own. Issues in the management of the psychiatry practice are described in a later section, but psychiatry appears to receive no discounts from the AEF or the administrative charges of Psychiatry Physicians, Inc. By contrast, the department of family medicine pays a discounted assessment for the academic enhancement fund, as well as a discounted assessment for university physicians' administrative costs.

While both the university hospital leadership and the leadership of the medical school acknowledge that they have not yet created a seamless system between them for dealing with payers, they nevertheless have a structure under the chancellor, which should enable them to continually improve their efforts in this regard. The chancellor serves as the chair of the board of trustees of the privatized university hospital. The chancellor, the dean, the director of the faculty practice plan, the head of the university hospital, the head of children's hospital, and the head of the Colorado Psychiatric Hospital (Dr. James Shore) meet on a weekly basis to focus on the clinical enterprise. Dr. Shore is also serving as acting vice chancellor during this period. The practice plan and the hospital have developed a separate 501(c)3 corporation to build the new ambulatory care center. The faculty practice plan is centralized; it learned from painful experience in the mid-1980s when its billing practices were subjected to an investigation by the state attorney general. However, the investigation has helped to focus the clinical departments and department heads on their responsibilities for documentation and oversight.

Recently the medical school altered its compensation guaranty for nontenured faculty and new appointees. The new compensation structure involves a guaranty of a salary targeted to levels of compensation of nonclinical faculty. A second component of compensation varies from year to year depending on prior year productivity. There are no discipline-specific standards of productivity within the faculty practice plan. Faculty signed their first capitation contract for state university employees in July 1995, but the vast majority of their contracts are for discounted fee-for-service plans.

There is a general recognition that the department of psychiatry enjoys relative advantages in being able to contract for bed costs and professional charges in a single consolidated fee because the chair of psychiatry also serves as the superintendent of the Colorado Psychiatric Hospital. The latter is a distinct operating entity within the University of Colorado Health Sciences Center, which will be elaborated on in a later section.

In addition to its commitment to public service, the University of Colorado School of Medicine has a proud tradition of research and tertiary care. It was one of the pioneering sites in organ transplant surgery. Until recently, however, medical students complained about a lack of commitment to education among the faculty. In the past 3 years, the undergraduate curriculum has been extensively reorganized to emphasize a longitudinal primary care course. The school has identified 375 primary care preceptors for each of 375 students. Each student is assigned to a primary care office for one-half day per week across a 3-year period. In this context, students have the opportunity to follow patients and families and to learn about the psychosocial aspects of patient care, including growth and development. Students participate in small group sessions once a month focusing on growth and development issues under the direction of a psychiatrist or psychologist.

The preclinical curriculum has been reorganized to be synchronous with developments in the longitudinal primary care experience. In the first year, students learn history taking and physical examination, along with organ system physiology and pathology. The second year emphasizes growth and development and the third year health policy and managed care. The school has received a number of grants to support this new educational initiative. Everyone that I spoke with in the medical school was highly enthusiastic about the changes in the curriculum. The chair of the department of family medicine expects that the undergraduate experiences of the university's students will force them to rethink the graduate medical education (GME) curriculum in family medicine because students are now better prepared for their residency.

Graduate medical education at the University of Colorado is the responsibility of the medical school rather than the teaching hospital. Each of the residency program directors serves as a member of the GME committee. The school provides interim evaluations to assist departments in anticipating issues in the external review process while strengthening GME overall in the institution. The university expects that there will be a substantial decrease in the number of fellows in the subspecialties of medicine and surgery, as well as an overall decrease in medical student interest. In several departments, efforts are already under way to replace a workforce previously made up of residents.

Among medical center leadership, the psychiatry department enjoys a high degree of respect. Over the past decade, Dr. James Shore (the department chair), has served at various times as acting hospital director, acting chancellor, and (currently) acting vice chancellor. Some other senior faculty in the department have also played highly important and visible roles in the medical center. Dr. Steven Dubovsky, the vice chair for clinical affairs, served as chair of the most recent dean's search committee. Dr. Michael Weissberg has played a major role in the committee overseeing curriculum reform in the school of medicine, as has

Dr. Robert Freedman in the interdepartmental neuroscience programs in the school of medicine.

Despite this position of influence within the medical center, and the presence of a rather large faculty, the clinical programs of the department are largely defined by the structure of the Colorado Psychiatric Hospital within the medical center and a relatively small consultation service to the university hospital and the Veterans Administration medical center (VAMC). The consultation service plays its most significant role in relationship to the liver transplant team. There is one half-time consultation psychiatrist (Dr. House) at the university hospital and two consultation psychiatrists at the VA. There is no overall oversight of psychosocial services within the medical center. The departments of family medicine and physical medicine and rehabilitation have their own teams of psychologists. The chair of family medicine spoke proudly of his team of mental health professionals, which includes psychology interns and graduate students from the University of Denver. A half-time psychiatrist serves as consultant to ambulatory care clinics in family medicine and general internal medicine, but her role was minimized by the chair of family medicine.

Within the past 6 years, all pediatric services of the university have been consolidated at Denver Children's Hospital. This arrangement has worked out extremely well for the department of pediatrics, whose clinical income and research support has grown substantially during this period (according to Dean Richard Krugman). However, it appears that the consolidation of pediatric services did not take adequate account of the needs and potential opportunities for child psychiatry in the planning and implementation effort. The child psychiatry educational programs are based at the Colorado Psychiatric Hospital, the Denver Children's Hospital, and other affiliated programs.

The Department of Psychiatry at the University of Colorado Health Sciences Center

Dr. James Shore became chair of the department of psychiatry and superintendent of the Colorado Psychiatric Hospital in 1985 following a long period of department chair vacancy. The first department chair

(Dr. Ebaugh) served from 1924 to 1953. His successor (Dr. Gaskill) served from 1953 to 1973. Dr. Herbert Pardes served as chair from 1975 to 1978, but because of his brief tenure the chair was mostly vacant between 1973 and 1985. During this period, the department developed a reputation as a center for psychoanalytic education consequent to the establishment of the Denver Psychoanalytic Institute as a partner and affiliate of the department of psychiatry in the early 1970s. Researchers, including several who had been recruited by Dr. Pardes, felt that their roles were marginal within the structure of the department of psychiatry. In the mid-1980s, prior to Dr. Shore's recruitment, efforts were made to merge the Colorado Psychiatric Hospital into the university hospital structure. Dr. Shore's recruitment aborted that process.

Before his arrival in Denver, Dr. Shore had a very distinguished career as professor and chair of the department of psychiatry at the University of Oregon, with research interests in community, social, and transcultural psychiatry (especially the mental health and general health care needs of Native Americans). As described by Dr. Shore, the department has an extremely broad mission that includes a substantial commitment to public psychiatry and the care of the indigent, to undergraduate and graduate medical education, and to the advancement of knowledge through an extremely wide-ranging portfolio of grant-supported research. In this context, it is difficult to identify a primary mission. Nevertheless, because of the strong tradition of state support for the Colorado Psychiatric Hospital in indigent care and in statewide GME for public service, we conclude that this department's primary mission is necessarily public service, but it has also been extraordinarily successful in developing first-class research and cutting-edge patient care programs.

The department is ranked second in the school in total research support from the National Institutes of Health (NIH). It is third in the country among departments of psychiatry in state-funded medical schools and within the top 10 of all departments of psychiatry in NIH research support. Its research programs are described in a later section (Research Programs). Consistent with the broad mission elaborated by Dr. Shore, the department has attempted to develop innovative approaches across the span of its clinical, research, public service, and educational activities. The culture within the department is extremely collegial. Lines of authority and responsibility are clearly delineated in the academic department and within the Colorado Psychiatric Hospital. A defined mentorship program for junior faculty assists them in career development and preparation for the promotion and tenure process. An annual scientific poster day for junior faculty highlights the importance of scholarship within the culture of this faculty. One is struck by the high degree of respect and commitment to excellence that exists across the broad range of departmental programs. In these times of crisis for academic psychiatry and academic medicine, in a community listed as among the most intensively impacted by managed care, the morale and level of understanding of departmental mission and individual responsibility are extremely high.

Clinical Activities

Over the past 6 years, some of the clinical programs of the Colorado Psychiatric Hospital and the department of psychiatry have been extensively reorganized to work more effectively with managed behavioral health care organizations. In 1993 the university acquired a nearby (failed) private psychiatric hospital to house the inpatient and continuing care programs of the Colorado Psychiatric Hospital. The 14-bed locked private psychiatric service had previously (in 1990) been divided into an 8-bed locked service and a 6-bed open service. Under the Alternatives Program, the average inpatient length of stay has declined to slightly more than 4 days from its 1989 level of 24.3 days. An emergency/crisis service was incorporated into the continuum of care. Staffing costs were reduced by 15%. Overall recidivism rates did not increase, but readmission rates were increased for patients with psychosis. The psychiatrists staffing the private psychiatric unit are full-time and voluntary faculty who have been organized into a group and are paid for their clinical service on a discounted basis. The unit has developed a collaborative approach to utilization review with managed behavioral health care organizations. Because the department is able to address both the facility and professional components in its contracts as the Colorado Psychiatric Hospital, it has been able to offer highly competitive case rates. The department has accepted a case rate of $2,700 per hospitalization with one of the behavioral health care companies, PRO Behavioral Health. In all, it has contracts with six of the behavioral health companies operating in the area, as well as a capitated contract for university employees that currently pays $13 per member per month (PMPM) for 15,000 covered lives. There is no indemnity business left for private inpatient services.

Residents have not been incorporated into the clinical programs of the managed behavioral health care service. However, they staff the other inpatient unit, which serves Medicare, Medicaid, and medically indigent patients. Residents also staff a traditional psychiatric outpatient service built around psychotherapy supervision. The clinic recently set up a separate medication clinic to accept referrals from elsewhere in the system (e.g., other departments in the medical school). The future of the traditional inpatient and outpatient services will be tied to decisions being made at the state level relative to the carving out of Medicaid. It is possible that the Colorado Psychiatric Hospital will have to develop a model of care similar to that developed in the Alternatives Program for the Medicaid carveout. There is likely to be intense competition for this patient population from Denver General Hospital and perhaps from other providers. Parenthetically, the Alternatives Program just breaks even at this time, despite the fact that the private attending psychiatrists in the group are not paid a salary by the department and they pay rent for their offices.

At this writing, the department has been able to craft a high-quality and cost-efficient clinical delivery system that is highly regarded by managed care organizations. However, the program does not generate surpluses that can be redistributed to the other components of the academic mission, and the clinical program has been dissected away from any educational function. As managed care impacts on services that have traditionally incorporated residents, the department will face a substantial challenge to its clinical and educational programs. The funding the department receives from the state for its educational, indigent care, and public-sector programs will need to continue if the department is to maintain its effectiveness across the span of its mission.

The structure of the relationship between the Colorado Psychiatric Hospital and the department of psychiatry enables Dr. Shore and his colleagues to address the most significant aspects of contract negotiation and to move toward the creation of joint ventures. They are currently involved in discussions with one company regarding potential services to corporations in Colorado for employee assistance activities. The faculty are able to maintain some entrepreneurialism while being guided by the raison d'être of their academic mission. By virtue of the structure of the Colorado Psychiatric Hospital, Dr. Shore is an independent participant at the table in discussions around the creation of Health Care Colorado (HCC), as in the creation of Colorado Access for indigent care. The Colorado Psychiatric Hospital also plans to partner with the Mental Health Corporation of Denver to carve out the mental health component of the health care programs for Medicaid recipients.

The Public Sector

There are two state hospitals in Colorado (Ft. Logan in Denver and Pueblo State Hospital in Pueblo, Colorado). There are also 17 comprehensive mental health centers and 5 specialty clinics focusing on the needs of special populations. The director of the state mental health program describes the relationship between the university and the department of mental health as "excellent" since the arrival of Dr. Shore. Prior to Dr. Shore's arrival, "the Department was training for private practice." The department of psychiatry hires all physicians working in the state hospitals under contract arrangements with the superintendent of each of the hospitals. The department of psychiatry collects 8% of the value of the contract for the costs of administration. The department has created a division of public-sector psychiatry that incorporates these faculty, as well as a major program devoted to services research. Because of the arrangement with the university, 70% of the full-time physicians in the state hospital system in Colorado are board certified. Dr. Shore regards the involvement by the department in public-sector psychiatry as "good citizenship." The state hospital system offers graduates of the University of Colorado program excellent employment opportunities. Some residents are able to supplement their annual salaries as trainees by committing to work in the public sector for 1 year in the middle of their training program. The state hospitals also serve as part of the educational experience for medical students, as locations for drug trials, and as clinical laboratories for the services research program.

The public sector is changing in Colorado, as it is changing in other states. Dr. Shore is chair of a commission looking at the future structure for the two state hospitals. A pilot study of a Medicaid carveout will ultimately be applied statewide, impacting on Denver and on the training programs within the Colorado Psychiatric Hospital. Dr. Barrett (the state mental health director) expects that there will be statewide capitation of Medicaid by 1997 or 1998 at a rate of $10 to $30 PMPM, depending on the Medicaid client population. The department of mental health has established criteria for required services based on five discrete levels of need. It has also established a performance indicator system that looks at consumer satisfaction, as well as change in functional status. A toll-free number to the office of consumer affairs to receive complaints from clients or providers has been established, as well as requirements for quality assurance within approved programs. The National Institute of Mental Health (NIMH) has created a research program to assess the effects of capitation on access to care, cost-effectiveness of service, and organizational issues. While the grant goes through the Berkeley Research Group, the services research programs at the university complement the service programs in the public sector. The department chair is clearly involved and committed to public-sector programs as a core part of the mission of the department of psychiatry.

Educational Programs

The department of psychiatry is responsible for 66 lecture hours and 33 seminar hours related to human behavior. In addition, the department provides 20 hours per year in the patient care segment of the first 2 years of the curriculum. There is a required 6-week clerkship that involves 4 students at the university site, 4 to 5 students at the Veterans Administration (VA) and 9 to 10 students per rotation at affiliated sites. The department offers 12 electives in the fourth year. Dr. Shore ranks the medical student education programs as most important, commencing with the programs in the first 2 years of the curriculum and then the clerkship. Residency education, primary care education, the education of other mental health professionals, and the reeducation of psychiatrists and other mental health professionals to better serve the needs of managed care were ranked in that order.

The chair of family medicine ranked the psychiatry clerkship, the psychiatric residency, and the education of other mental health professionals as the top three in importance, followed by preclinical course teaching, primary care education, the continuing education of professionals in practice and history, and physical examination teaching. In general, psychiatry did not rank very highly in his view relative to primary care education and the education of medical students in the introduction to patient care. In the family medicine chair's view, these areas should be taught by primary care physicians rather than psychiatrists.

The dean of the medical school rated the psychiatry clerkship and other psychiatry teaching in the first 2 years as most important, followed by the psychiatry residency, primary care education, the education of other mental health professionals, and the continuing education of psychiatrists and other mental health professionals relative to managed care. The commitment of the department of psychiatry to medical student teaching, as emphasized by Dr. Shore and by the dean, is borne out by the fact that 6% of the school's graduates are going into psychiatry, a number far higher than the national average. In addition, the director of the medical student education program, Dr. Michael Weissberg, was named by the medical students as the best basic science teacher for the second-year course.

The residency training program currently has 45 residents. In academic year 1994–1995, there were 15 postgraduate year (PGY) II residents. This number was reduced to 12 in academic year 1995–1996, a figure that will either remain at 12 or decline further to 10 residents per year. Dr. House (the residency program director) projects that the next 5 years in the training program will emphasize briefer psychotherapies, more effective medication management, more effective consultation to other disciplines, more effective integration with managed care systems, better training in substance abuse, and better integration of new technologies into practice. He expects that the training program will continue to downsize, as will the training programs for other mental health disciplines. He sees great employment opportunities for university graduates in rural areas of the Rocky Mountains and the Midwest, as well as in the public sector.

As it now stands, the training program appears to be fairly standard. In the internship year, residents spend 2 months on neurology, 4 months on internal medicine, 1 month in the medical-surgical emergency department, 1 month in the psychiatric emergency department, 2 months on addiction services (1 month detoxification and 1 month addiction rehabilitation), 1 month on adolescence psychiatry, and 1 month of a selective experience. The second year involves three inpatient rotations for all residents, including 4 months at the VA, 4 months at Colorado Psychiatric Hospital, and 4 months at Denver General Hospital. The third year involves a longitudinal sequence of 2 to 3 hours per day on a consultation-liaison service and the remainder of the time in adult and child outpatient care.

As described previously, the outpatient experience at the Colorado Psychiatric Hospital appears to be a traditional psychotherapy educational experience. The fourth year involves a variety of electives, 10 hours per week in the outpatient department and 1 day a week at a community mental health center. At the May 1995 meeting of the American Psychiatric Association, Dr. Shore made a proposal for the creation of a primary care track within psychiatry. He argued that psychiatrists need to be able to provide basic primary medical care for seriously mentally ill patients who do not have adequate access to general health care. He proposed a new curricular model and a track that would include training for diagnostic and primary care skills for psychiatrists, suggesting that such a plan would be possible within current accreditation requirements of the residency review committee (RRC). Residents electing this track would receive primary care training throughout their residency. Dr. Shore's proposal is quite specific. The primary care psychiatrists would serve as the general physician and psychiatrist for an assigned caseload within the state public sector or the VA. The primary care would focus principally on stable and noncomplex medical problems. The arguments in the paper are well articulated, and Dr. Shore has begun to implement the experience with selected residency in their fourth year of training.

Parenthetically, the chair of the department of family medicine, Dr. Larry Green, does not believe that a psychiatrist can perform the functions of a primary care physician as outlined by Dr. Shore. While Dr. Shore and his colleagues seem enthusiastic about the possibilities of primary care education for psychiatrists, they will need to work hard to establish the type of partnership that would make collaborative education possible with their sister departments in primary care at Colorado.

Finally, the department supports postresidency training fellowships in forensic psychiatry and addiction psychiatry and postdoctoral research training in a number of areas. The child psychiatry training program is part of the Colorado Psychiatric Hospital and has links to Denver Children's Hospital. There are no immediate plans to change these training programs or to add an additional fellowship in geriatric psychiatry.

Relationship With the Department of Veterans Affairs

The Denver Veterans Administration (VA) Hospital programs in psychiatry are tied to the educational, research, and clinical programs of the department at the university in a number of ways. The VA hospital shares the health center campus. The consultation-liaison service operates in a unified fashion between the university hospital and the VA hospital. All residents rotate through the inpatient and addiction rehabilitation services at the VA, and the VA service educates a substantial percentage of medical students during the psychiatry clerkship. During the tenure of Dr. Herbert Pardes in the mid-1970s, Dr. Robert Freedman was recruited to develop a research program in the department of psychiatry at the VA hospital. However, until recently, VA psychiatry was largely staffed by part-time clinicians with no research interests. In this regard, the service was quite different from the departments of medicine and surgery.

Dr. Martin Reite, a longtime psychiatric researcher in the department, was selected as chief of psychiatry at the VA in October 1994. He is committed to staffing the VA service with full-time academic psychiatrists. By his report, the VA leadership at Denver is strongly committed to the traditional tripartite mission of patient care, education, and research.

The VA psychiatry service is responsible for 106 beds, including 16 inpatient adult psychiatry (40 locked, 20 open), 30 long-term beds for the treatment of posttraumatic stress disorder (PTSD), and 30 beds devoted to the treatment of substance abuse. There are presently 18.75 positions for psychiatrists. This number may be cut by one to two positions over the next few years, and there is likely to be a cut in inpatient beds; the consolidation of mental health disciplines (social work, psychology, and psychiatry) within the VA should make for a smoother clinical operation. Nevertheless, Dr. Reite pointed out to me that 80% of a full-time psychiatrist's time is devoted to clinical work in the VA, whereas comparable figures in surgery are 67% and in medicine 49%. Thus, a disproportionate allocation of slots relative to clinical work exists for this VA, as for other hospitals in the VA system. Moreover, many of the medical-surgical patients are being hospitalized for non-service-connected disorders, whereas the mental health disciplines are only able to work with service-connected problems.

In spite of the relative disadvantages facing psychiatry in the VA system (compared with medicine), Dr. Reite was upbeat about the prospects for the psychiatry service at Denver. As he pointed out, the previous reliance on part-time clinicians means that he can make selective cuts and that his part-time clinicians can spend all of their time at the VA in clinical activity. He is therefore able to provide some protected time for junior faculty to enable them to develop as researchers and academicians during their clinical work. The VA serves as the clinical base for the schizophrenia research center funded by NIMH, as well as for the research center funded by the VA.

Research Programs

In academic year 1995–1996, the department of psychiatry generated more than $13 million a year in extramural grant support, including $10.2 million from the federal government and $1.8 million from the corporate sector. The research programs are wide-ranging, including basic studies on neuroembryogenesis in the chick, studies of cellular transplantation in brain, stress and development in primates, studies using magnetoencepholography and brain imaging in humans, population genetics, clinical research, population-based studies in Native Americans and Alaskans, and services research on the chronically and severely mentally ill. There is also a model interuniversity program for studies in early infant development headed by the distinguished research child psychiatrist, Dr. Robert Emde.

The research portfolio includes separately funded NIMH and VA center grants for schizophrenia research, a major program of research on the relationship between conduct disorder and substance use in drug-abusing youth, and the National Center for American Indian and Alaskan

Native Mental Health Research. The latter also receives major funding from the Robert Wood Johnson Foundation. Important collaborative efforts include the Rocky Mountain Center for Sensor Technology, the early developmental studies supported by the NIMH and MacArthur Foundation, and strong collaborations with the University of Utah department of genetics and the Karolinska Institute in Sweden (with the Schizophrenia Center). The work of the schizophrenia research center was recently strengthened by a major grant from a venture capitalist.

Dr. Robert Freedman serves as vice chair for research. He sees his role as adviser to Dr. Shore and (along with other senior faculty) as mentor to junior faculty. His own career at Colorado has been instructive. He was recruited to a full-time position at the Denver Veterans Administration Medical Center out of his residency at the University of Chicago by Dr. Herbert Pardes. Shortly after his arrival, Dr. Pardes left to become director of the NIMH. With the assistance of colleagues in the department of pharmacology and the alcohol research center (funded by the National Institute on Alcohol Abuse and Alcoholism), Dr. Freedman was able to gain protected time and to propel his research. The group in pharmacology also provided the intellectual stimulation that he needed during the years prior to Dr. Shore's arrival (1978–1985). He feels that it is his and Dr. Shore's responsibility to engage new faculty in a process of "informed consent" to recognize that they need to become involved in supported research in order to secure protected time for their scholarly work. Dr. Freedman, Dr. Shore, and their colleagues have been extremely supportive to faculty-development efforts (see earlier section).

The research programs of the department benefit substantially from the presence of an NIMH-funded clinical research center (CRC) at the university, functional magnetic resonance imaging (MRI), single photon emission computerized tomography (SPECT), a strong behavioral genetics program at the university, basic neuroscientists through a number of basic science departments at the health sciences campus, and a strong biostatistics program at the university. There is also a strong epidemiology program at the National Center for American Indian and Alaskan Native Mental Health Research in the department of psychiatry.

The University of Colorado does not have a positron-emission tomography (PET) imaging program, and there are no small grants for

pilot research from the university. The major challenge facing Dr. Freedman will be how to maintain and strengthen a research infrastructure
that is becoming increasingly oriented to basic science. The university
needs to be able to recruit basic scientists who are on the cutting-edge
of their research fields. Increasingly, research in many places is non-
departmental. The interdepartmental neuroscience program at the university has been somewhat hampered by the recruitment of strong department chairs. The school itself is divided between those who want
to create a basic neurobiology program and those who want a program
that emphasizes the clinical neurosciences. Research space and new faculty represent a critical need. Psychiatry will need a basic molecular and
cellular neurobiology program oriented to behavior. Dr. Freedman
served as chair of the search committee for a head of the neuroscience
program at the university, but a lack of resolution of critical governance
and funding questions thwarted their recruitment effort. The challenge
will be to move this process to its conclusion and to keep psychiatry
involved in the discussions on the future infrastructure for genetics,
molecular and cellular neurobiology, and brain imaging.

In meetings with Dr. Freedman, Dr. Shore, Dr. Spero Manson (the
head of the National Center for American Indian and Alaskan Native
Mental Health Research), and members of the department of psychiatry
executive committee, it is obvious that the faculty under Dr. Shore's
direction have a clear vision of the future of their major research programs and an understanding of the issues that need to be addressed.

Summary

Under the leadership of Dr. James Shore and a talented faculty, the
University of Colorado department of psychiatry has developed a broad
array of strengths that should enable it to cope effectively with the crisis
facing academic psychiatry. Dr. Shore and his senior colleagues continue
to play extremely important roles within the school of medicine and in
relationship to the public sector. Morale among the faculty is excellent,
and there is a deep commitment to career development among younger
faculty. Despite the fact that only 8% of faculty salaries comes from the
university, and a lean, managed care–friendly clinical program cannot

provide significant support for the academic mission, the department has pulled together broadly based sources of federal, state, foundation, and corporate support for its academic mission. Research centers play an important role in the life of the department and in the career development of young faculty; Colorado's research effort is truly impressive. The educational programs of the department appear to be thriving, with a full residency class and impressive interest in psychiatry among the medical school graduates.

Because of the unique structure and funding of the Colorado Psychiatric Hospital and its relationship to the department of psychiatry, Dr. Shore is in an unusually good position to craft programs that serve the needs of managed care corporations and that can bring together the public-sector, Medicare, and insured patients in a single, coherent service delivery system.

There are some problem areas of which the department and the medical center appear to be aware. The Denver Children's Hospital has seemingly made little effort to incorporate the clinical, educational, and research programs important to child psychiatry. The Colorado Psychiatric Hospital will have difficulty mobilizing all of the resources on its own for the development of a full academic effort in child psychiatry without a closer degree of collaboration with Denver Children's Hospital. Within the health sciences center, there is an awareness that some of the most significant new managed care contracts (e.g., for CHAMPUS) will end up excluding psychiatry at this juncture because of the nature of the multistate arrangements and the fact that behavioral health care has already been carved out by prior agreement. In the future, the programs at the Colorado Psychiatric Hospital need to be incorporated into the overall contractual effort.

Within the health sciences center, there is only selective penetration by the consultation-liaison service, principally in the liver transplant program and (to an underappreciated degree) in primary care ambulatory settings. The lack of a fuller collaboration with one of the primary care departments may inhibit the psychiatry department's vision to create a primary care–psychiatry track within its residency program. Within the department itself, the residency training program has not been incorporated into the managed care clinical activities, and the training program may be under great pressure when the behavioral health services for Medicaid patients in Denver come under managed care. The current managed care unit in the department is under economic pressure and generates no surplus that can be applied to the academic mission. The department is critically dependent on continued state support for the Colorado Psychiatric Hospital in its mission of indigent care, education, and research.

The Department of Psychiatry at the University of Louisville

Roger E. Meyer, M.D.

I visited the University of Louisville department of psychiatry and the school of medicine on December 6–7, 1995. I had meetings with Dr. Allan Tasman (department of psychiatry chair), Dr. Donald Kmetz (vice president for health affairs and dean of the school of medicine), Dr. Larry Cook (chair of the Medical School Practice Association and chair of the department of pediatrics), Dr. Richard Redinger (chair of the department of medicine), Dr. Richard Clover (chair of the department of family and community medicine), and Dr. Gordon Strauss (director of the psychiatry residency training program). I also met with the medical director of a local managed behavioral health company, Dr. Robert Atkins of ClearSprings. I was unable to meet with Mr. Ronald Hytoff, president and chief executive officer of the University of Louisville Hospital, because the hospital was undergoing a change in management from Columbia/HCA to a new governing coalition (see later section).

General Environment

The University of Louisville Medical School is one of two state-supported medical schools in Kentucky. It is part of a state university that has historically had a relatively small research budget. The campus of the medical school serves as a regional tertiary care center, with the principal teaching hospitals adjacent to each other. These hospitals include the children's hospital (which is linked to the Alliant Hospital System), the Norton Hospital (Alliant Hospital system), Jewish Hospital, and the University of Louisville Hospital. The local Department of Veterans Affairs hospital is an approximately 10-minute drive from this site. Dr. Donald Kmetz has been vice president and dean for many years and (by his report) enjoys an excellent relationship with the parent university.

Dr. Kmetz was responsible for negotiating the original leasing arrangement of the University of Louisville Hospital to the Humana Corporation. Under the original terms of the lease contract, 20% of the profits of the hospital were to be turned over to the school of medicine. Vice President Kmetz indicated that the university's expected return did not materialize over the course of the contract because of the high management fee charged by Humana. The experience of this university should be instructive to other academic medical centers currently considering arrangements with for-profit hospital corporations.

The lease contract was originally developed in 1983. When Humana decided to leave the hospital business to focus its efforts on managed care, it sold its hospitals to the corporation that eventually became Columbia/HCA. Because the terms of the lease arrangement required the parent corporation to keep its headquarters in Louisville, the decision by Columbia/HCA to relocate its headquarters to Nashville abrogated the lease. Columbia/HCA did bid for the successor contract, offering 50% of the "profits." Alliant and Jewish Hospitals joined together to create a new corporation, University Medical Center, Inc., to manage the University of Louisville Hospital. They guaranteed $33 million over the first 3 years of the contract to the school of medicine. The arrangement also offers the possibility of greater collaboration among the medical school and its logical clinical partners. Jewish Hospital is the premier heart and transplant center in the region. Alliant Hospital dominates oncology and pediatric care. The university hospital has a highly regarded trauma program.

Given the concentration of beds at the medical school site, the new arrangement should allow these institutions to prepare for the future

impact of managed care on bed occupancy. At this writing, Louisville
has not experienced a significant impact from managed care, so bed
occupancy is quite high. While overall managed care represents an insignificant portion of the current market, a number of managed behavioral health companies are competing for behavioral health carveouts.
The companies receive capitated payments and pay individual providers
on a discounted fee-for-service basis. The per member per month
(PMPM) rate received by these companies varies between $2.00 and
$2.50. I met with Dr. Robert Atkins, the medical director of Clear-
Springs, a managed behavioral health company owned by Alliant and
Baptist Hospitals. The company is responsible for 165,000 covered lives
and has contracts with 56 psychiatrists and a total of 200 clinicians
statewide in Kentucky, Southern Indiana, Ohio, and West Virginia. Dr.
Atkins indicates that the goals of the parent corporation are to keep the
psychiatric beds filled and that this expectation runs counter to the real
possibilities of a managed behavioral health company. At the present
time, there is no relationship between the academic department of psychiatry and ClearSprings because Dr. Tasman believes that the discounted fee-for-service rate is not sufficient. Nevertheless, the recent
alliance of the medical school with Alliant (as well as Jewish Hospital),
could lead to potential new collaborations between the university department of psychiatry and the managed care subsidiary of Alliant
(ClearSprings).

The Department of Psychiatry

Dr. Allan Tasman became the chair of the department of psychiatry in
1991 following the retirement of the previous longtime chair, Dr. John
Schwab. Dr. Tasman had a distinguished prior career as a residency
training director, as well as a widely acknowledged national leadership
role in academic psychiatry and the American Psychiatric Association.
He describes the primary mission of his department as 1) residency
education, 2) medical student education, 3) clinical service to under-
served populations, and 4) research. He has clearly configured the effort
and future of the department in these directions.

The residency program appears to be thriving. The medical students at the university account for approximately half of the residents in the graduate medical education (GME) program, and Dr. Tasman believes that this number is a function of the success of the medical student education programs. Dr. Tasman has been involved in major negotiations with the State Department of Mental Health to establish a holding bed unit at the University of Louisville Hospital and to transfer salary support for lines for psychiatrists at the local state hospital to the university budget. He has forged an effective collaboration with the local community mental health center leadership and has a clear vision for a coordinated public-sector psychiatry program linked to the university department.

Education

The department of psychiatry offers 64 lecture hours in behavioral science, a 6-week required clerkship, a residency program with 42 residents (including 4 child fellows) and a consultation-liaison fellowship. There are currently 11 postgraduate year (PGY) II residents in the program. There might be 10 such residents in the year 2000.

As one might expect, Dr. Tasman lists the psychiatric residency training program as the most important educational activity in the department, followed by the psychiatry clerkship and primary care education, with relatively low priority for the reeducation of psychiatrists and other mental health professionals to work in managed care settings. The priorities of the dean emphasized psychiatry's role in primary care education, the psychiatry clerkship, the psychiatry residency, and the reeducation of psychiatrists to better serve managed care. It was of interest that none of the three chairs of the primary care departments listed primary care education as the most important priority in psychiatric education. The representative of managed care, Dr. Atkins of ClearSprings, placed the highest priority on psychiatric residency education, with the education of primary care physicians and other mental health professionals as other high priorities. In his view, the department was not educating residents for managed care practice. The five most critical skills for psychiatrists, according to Dr. Atkins, are 1) enhanced consultant skills "without sounding like psychiatrists," 2) choice of the treatment model that will produce the outcome desired by the patient,

3) team leadership skills, 4) quantitative skills measuring the outcome of psychiatric practice, and 5) therapeutic alliance ability.

Despite Dr. Atkins's critique, the skills identified by Dr. Tasman and his training director were not far from those identified by Dr. Atkins. Dr. Tasman emphasized the five skills as follows: 1) diagnosis (including imaging and other sophisticated technology), 2) somatic interventions (including possible future gene therapy), 3) knowledge of psychotherapeutic interventions, 4) team leadership across a continuum of care, and 5) administration. The training director, Dr. Strauss, emphasized 1) careful interviewing and assessment beyond a diagnosis, 2) broad knowledge about therapeutic modalities that work, 3) curiosity about meaning in the doctor-patient relationship, 4) knowledge of group and organizational processes leading to effective team and systems leadership, and 5) knowledge of clinically relevant neuroscience.

The residency program is already in transition, with the implementation of a "Firm Model" at the Veterans Administration (VA) and interest at Norton Hospital (part of the Alliant system) in a similar arrangement. The development of the Firm Model by site was not as clear to me as the overall residency program changes at Dartmouth. Both Dr. Tasman and Dr. Strauss recognize that a consolidation of program sites is necessary since residents are currently covering four emergency rooms at the same time. The consolidation of the public-sector system (as described previously) should facilitate a more rational allocation of residents to service areas. The Firm Model, if implemented across the training program, should begin to meet the needs of managed care in the area. As a rural state with three modest-sized metropolitan areas, Kentucky probably does not have a great surplus of psychiatrists. Nevertheless, there has been no active planning among the major training programs to determine actual workforce needs.

The significant educational innovation currently under way at the medical school involves the development of a continuous 24-week primary care sequence in the third year. This plan is presenting some logistical problems for the department of psychiatry and its clerkship. Dr. Tasman views the new emphasis on primary care as an opportunity for the department to become more actively involved in teaching primary care settings to medical students and primary care residents. The 24-week sequence is to begin with the incoming third-year class, in which 12 medical students will function in an interdisciplinary clinic with physicians and physician extenders. As of December 1995, there was still no site identified for the clinic or funds for faculty. The planning for this initiative came from an initial Robert Wood Johnson Foundation grant, but the implementation phase was not funded. It appears that the dean may be able to use some of the new dollars from the lease of the hospital to commit to this effort, but there is also interest in using the funds to create a health maintenance organization (HMO) to serve the Medicaid population.

The department of psychiatry is involved in the education of primary care physicians in family medicine, pediatrics, and internal medicine using focused case consultations in the primary care setting and rotation of primary care (family medicine) residents on psychiatry services and in lectures and seminars by psychiatry faculty in the primary care departments. The program is most active in family medicine, where residents have a 4-week rotation, generally in an ambulatory setting. Internal medicine has shown interest in some type of rotation for general internists, and pediatrics offers rotations to child psychiatry on an elective basis. The new chair of family medicine seemed genuinely enthusiastic about collaborative educational programs with the department of psychiatry, which would dovetail nicely with the interests in the department of psychiatry in developing a behavioral medicine initiative, as well as innovative approaches to the delivery of primary care and mental health services elaborated by the training director in psychiatry. All parties showed reasonable consensus about the skills primary care physicians should have regarding diagnosis and treatment of mental and addictive disorders.

Clinical Service

The department has not reconfigured its services to deal with managed care and appears to see its interest more clearly tied to the public sector (as described earlier). The two state medical schools plan to become involved in a state managed care program for Medicaid recipients and in the creation of an HMO. A consultant is working with the Medical School Practice Association to prepare members to work with this Medicaid-based HMO. The school plans to use disproportionate share

(DISH) dollars to set up the HMO. Because behavioral health services will be carved out in this arrangement, it is not clear to other departments how psychiatry can effectively become involved (apart from its own efforts with the public sector). Its role needs to be clarified and developed.

The Faculty Practice Association is highly decentralized. There is a 3.45% tax on individual net income from professional services. Accountability for oversight rests with the department chair. There is also a separate departmental tax on individual faculty members' billings to create academic enhancement funds within the clinical department. Three separate practice corporations within the department of psychiatry were inherited by the current chair. The overall system does not appear to be ready for the impact of managed care, or even the impact of the proposed HMO for Medicaid patients. The head of the practice plan, Dr. Cook, acknowledges that faculty are resistant to any centralized control. The chairs meet on a bimonthly basis to discuss issues of practice management. The new arrangement with Alliant and Jewish Hospitals, coupled with the creation of the HMO, should produce tremendous pressures for change within the faculty practice environment.

Since 1991, the department has not been in a deficit situation. University support has been stable at approximately $1.4 million per year. Clinical income has grown slowly and currently amounts to approximately $2.5 million per year. The department's 1995–96 budget was $5.8 million. There are presently nine tenured professors, eight tenured and five nontenured associate professors, and seven nontenured assistant professors who are psychiatrists in the department. There are three tenured nonpsychiatrist professors, two tenured nonpsychiatrist associate professors, and five nontenured nonpsychiatrist assistant professors in the department. Dr. Tasman anticipates some growth in nontenured assistant professorships and tenured full professorships (psychiatrists) as a consequence of the anticipated contract with the State Department of Mental Health.

There is no tradition of significant voluntary faculty teaching in the Louisville area, although the department anticipates a significant increase in voluntarism among its recent graduates. The absence of a strong network of voluntary faculty limits the department's ability to provide leadership in networking of nonpsychiatrists and psychiatrists to serve behavioral health carveouts.

The department clearly sees its future in relationship to linkages with the public sector and an excellent relationship with the VA under new psychiatry leadership at the institution. The department's upbeat assessment of the VA contrasted with the negative assessment of the VA by the department of medicine, which is suffering from a projected cutback in support at the institution.

Research

The psychiatry department's efforts to support a promising young investigator recruited from NIH is instructive. A laboratory was created and 3 years of funding were provided by the department as part of the recruitment package that had been offered by the dean to Dr. Tasman. The program has not successfully competed for outside grants but has received one small grant from a local foundation. There is no substantial basic neuroscience program in the medical school, and the weakness in the department of neurology was highlighted by the dean. The latter had considered combining the departments of psychiatry, neurology, and neurosurgery into a clinical neuroscience program but was discouraged from doing so by outside consultants. There is no infrastructure for neuroscience research at the University of Louisville, which meant that the young investigator was relatively isolated. It appears that, to be successful, he would have had to collaborate with investigators at other universities.

More recently, Dr. Tasman has been focusing on efforts to secure foundation support to create a behavioral medicine institute. This attempt seems to dovetail nicely with the interests in the medical school in strengthening the primary care delivery system. Securing foundation support, along with the efforts under way with the state system, define the potential for the department in the near and intermediate future. The University of Louisville practice environment, which has no cap on physician income and a highly decentralized administrative structure, has served to limit the development of a significant research infrastructure at this medical school. The absence of a research tradition should present no barrier to directing faculty efforts to increase clinical productivity. However, the absence of an accountable structure for the practice environment will challenge the leadership of the institution as it seeks to deal with the arrival of managed care. The combined strengths of the Alliant and Jewish Hospitals, in conjunction with the university, offer a real opportunity to protect the tertiary care and educational missions of this medical school and its teaching hospitals. Psychiatry should do well in this environment if support from the public sector can be secured and good relationships with the primary care departments maintained.

Summary

The department of psychiatry at the University of Louisville appears to be fulfilling its defined mission. It is doing well in its medical student and residency education programs, and it appears to have a promising future in the development of educational programs and behavioral medicine collaborations with the department of family medicine. It is clearly focusing the future of its patient care activities on the linkages with the public sector. The decentralized practice arrangements give the chair considerable latitude in determining how to direct the practice activities of the department. At the same time, the weak structure of the faculty practice plan represents something of an Achilles' heel for the future of the medical center as it deals with managed care.

The Department of Psychiatry at Dartmouth–Hitchcock Medical Center

Roger E. Meyer, M.D.

I visited the department of psychiatry at the Dartmouth-Hitchcock Medical Center on August 26–27, 1996. I met with Mr. James Varnum (president of the Mary Hitchcock Memorial Hospital), Mr. John Collins (executive vice president of the Lahey-Hitchcock Clinic), Dr. Andrew Wallace and Dr. William Culp (dean and the associate dean, respectively, for academic affairs at the Dartmouth Medical School), Mr. Gary DeGasta (director of the affiliated Veterans Administration [VA] medical center at White River Junction in Vermont), and Mr. Jesse Turner (president and chief executive officer of West Central Services). I also met with Dr. Harold Sox (chair of the department of medicine), who is a well-recognized national leader in general internal medicine and primary care. Within the department of psychiatry, I met with Dr. Peter Silberfarb (chair), Mr. David Budlong (administrative director of the department), Dr. Robert Vidaver (vice chair and medical director of the New Hampshire Hospital), Dr. Leighton Huey (vice chair and medical director of the department of psychiatry), and Dr. Ronald Green (director of education and training).

Dartmouth Medical School

Dartmouth Medical School's roots reach into the eighteenth century, although it was only reborn as a 4-year medical school in the early 1970s. It functions as one of the corporate entity components of the Dartmouth-Hitchcock Medical Center, which also includes the Mary Hitchcock Memorial Hospital, the Lebanon division of the Lahey-Hitchcock Clinic, and the Veterans Administration medical center at White River Junction in Vermont. The Lahey-Hitchcock Clinic (consisting of the merger of the Lahey Clinic in Burlington, Massachusetts, and the Hitchcock Clinic and its multiple practice sites and satellites in southern New Hampshire) also owns the Matthew Thornton Health Plan, a health maintenance organization (HMO) in Nashua, New Hampshire. The Mary Hitchcock Memorial Hospital is the anchor hospital for a multihospital system called the Hitchcock Alliance.

The structure that has evolved over the past 70 years appears to be unique among academic health centers. For example, there is no executive for the Dartmouth-Hitchcock Medical Center. The Dartmouth-Hitchcock Medical Center board of trustees has no direct control over the budgets of its four components. Each of the principal entities has its own separate board of trustees. In the past few years, there has been some effort to provide overlap in membership of the boards of trustees for the clinic and the hospital. The dean of the school of medicine serves ex officio on both boards. The clinic and the hospital both contribute funds to support the school of medicine.

The financial arrangements are reviewed every 5 years. The clinic pays approximately 2.5% of revenue as a dean's tax. The hospital transfers cash payments to the school for direct support of house staff, as well as some teaching costs. In general, support for clinical department heads comes from the hospital, the clinic, and the school. The clinic, the hospital, and a significant portion of the medical school relocated to a brand-new campus in Lebanon, New Hampshire, in 1991. Facilities management for this site is under the direction of the hospital. Managed care activities for the Lebanon/Hanover, New Hampshire, area are negotiated through a single contracts office. There is also a single office dealing with information services for the clinical entities in this region. At this writing, managed care has been a less significant factor in this region than in the southern part of the state. However, this fact has begun to change in ways that are already impacting on hospital census and revenue (see later section).

The distinct and interdependent histories of the medical school, the clinic, and the hospital are of interest. The hospital was founded near the end of the last century. The school of medicine granted degrees (M.D.) until the publication of the Flexner Report, when it became a 2-year school focusing on preclinical education. Students then transferred to medical schools in urban centers to complete their medical education. The Hitchcock Clinic began in the 1920s under the leadership of Dr. John Bowler, who had come back to Hanover following training at the Mayo Clinic. Dr. Bowler persuaded four colleagues to join him in creating a group practice in which income was pooled and income from higher-earning surgical specialties could be used to support lower-earning disciplines, to subsidize the hospital, and to support medical education. This multispecialty group philosophy has continued, so that at equal academic rank, no individual can earn more than twice the salary of the lowest-paid medical specialist (according to Mr. John Collins, the executive vice president of Lahey-Hitchcock Clinic).

When the medical school again became a full M.D.-granting program in the 1970s, the medical staff of the clinic served as its clinical faculty. With the founding of the 4-year medical school, two clinical departments were created outside of the clinic structure, reporting directly to the dean. The department of community and family medicine was created, and a department of psychiatry was organized out of the division of psychiatry within the department of internal medicine at the clinic. The unique reporting relationship for psychiatry within this structure has enabled the department to develop opportunities that might have been difficult to implement within the traditional multispecialty group practice structure, while it has also created occasional problems relating to the planning and implementation of psychiatric and behavioral health services within the clinic and the hospital. These issues are elaborated further in the section dealing specifically with psychiatry.

Commencing in the early 1980s, the Hitchcock Clinic and the Mary Hitchcock Hospital embarked on discrete strategies, the clinic focusing on a "Southern Strategy." The southern part of the state included a number of strong hospitals and practices, and the most southern portions of the state were culturally linked to the Boston metropolitan area. Indeed, approximately 75,000 New Hampshire citizens and 125,000 of their dependents are employed in Massachusetts. The hospital crafted its strategy around the Hitchcock Alliance, linking a number of smaller hospitals in the less-populous northern part of the state to the Mary Hitchcock Memorial Hospital.

In 1984 the clinic acquired a six-member group practice in Manchester, New Hampshire, 65 miles southeast of the clinic. In 1985 it purchased an 18-member primary care practice in Concord, New Hampshire, and in 1994 the Keene Clinic joined the Hitchcock Clinic, adding 51 additional physicians. Between 1989 and 1994 the clinic increased the number of salaried physicians by 76% and added 18 major satellite centers housing two- to five-person practices, along with 23 outreach programs. In 1984 the clinic also began a partnership with the Matthew Thornton Health Plan in Nashua, New Hampshire; the HMO was then acquired by the clinic in 1989. Financing for additional growth came from the Hitchcock Clinic and the Mary Hitchcock Hospital. It is estimated that the HMO went from a net worth of negative $977,000 in 1989 to a positive value of $33 million in 1994.

Since 1994 the clinic has effected a merger with the Lahey Clinic in Burlington, Massachusetts, creating the Lahey-Hitchcock Clinic. These two nonprofit multispecialty practices have combined revenues of $700 million per year. The HMO's revenue is $200 million per year, and the revenue of the hospital is $220 million per year. At the Lahey Clinic site, most clinical activity is performed on a discounted fee-for-service basis. In southern New Hampshire, 60% of the clinic's revenue is on a capitated basis. In the northern region (with Lebanon and Hanover, New Hampshire, as the core), less than 5% of the clinic's revenue is on a capitated basis. In the recent past, the clinic has made strategic efforts to link up with the Harvard Community Health Plan (now the Harvard Pilgrim Health Plan), but these efforts have not been fruitful.

The Hitchcock Alliance has its own overall strategic plan linking the Mary Hitchcock Hospital to six hospitals and one community mental health center. To craft a network strategy, the hospital and its affiliated hospitals created a holding company whose chief executive officer is also the chief executive officer of Mary Hitchcock Hospital. Efforts are being made to allow local control of the separate facilities within this structure. The Mary Hitchcock Hospital has reduced average lengths of stay to less than 5 days and has developed partial hospital and transitional bed capacity for medical-surgical and psychiatric patients. The hospital chief executive officer is especially proud of the continuous quality improvement program developed by a team recruited from the Hospital Corporation of America (HCA).

At this writing, the hospital has decreased the number of staffed beds from 420 to 350. The census when I visited was under 300 patients. Only 8% of the hospital's patient mix is managed care, and little is capitated care. The hospital strategy for the northern part of the state has not included purchase of practices. The strengths of the decentralized system of governance of the Dartmouth-Hitchcock Medical Center have served to position the clinical delivery systems reasonably well. Without the center's efforts, the small population base around the Lebanon, New Hampshire, site would be insufficient to maintain an adequate clinical volume. Within the decentralized structure, Dartmouth Medical School is clearly the smallest financial component. The dean of Dartmouth Medical School, Dr. Andrew Wallace, described a generally favorable relationship among the entities of the Dartmouth-Hitchcock Medical Center, even as he anticipated that this year's budget would be the same as last year's.[1]

The regional uniqueness of the Dartmouth-Hitchcock Medical Cen-

---

[1] While the dean, Mr. Collins, and Mr. Varnum all highlighted the strengths of the decentralized system, there were some problems in implementing different strategies. For example, the entrepreneurially driven programs of the clinic in the southern region appear to be disconnected from the ambulatory educational needs of the school of medicine. The latter has not been involved in planning around these practices relative to its significant need for ambulatory educational sites. Moreover, within the newly merged Lahey-Hitchcock Clinic, the Lahey Clinic site continues to be a major locus for undergraduate medical student education at Tufts Medical School. It does not appear that the medical school and the leadership of the Lahey-Hitchcock Clinic have begun to address the rich possibilities of a new clinical affiliation as it might apply to medical student education for Dartmouth Medical School. These apparent shortcomings can be corrected over time; some of the most interesting have occurred in relationship to the department of psychiatry at Dartmouth and the separate behavioral health strategies of the Lahey-Hitchcock Clinic and the Hitchcock Alliance. Some resolution of the latter issues could help to strengthen intersecting strategies for the de facto partners of the Dartmouth-Hitchcock Medical Center.

ter has enabled the school to play a leadership role in rural health and primary care education, but it has limited the opportunities in certain specialties such as obstetrics/gynecology and emergency medicine. The board of overseers for the medical school is separate from the Dartmouth board of trustees, which has a subcommittee for the medical school. There is some overlap between the membership of the board of overseers and this subcommittee of Dartmouth College trustees. The dean reports to the provost on academic issues and to the president of Dartmouth College on strategic issues. In 1992–1993, the dean headed a strategic planning process for the Dartmouth-Hitchcock Medical Center that covered clinical activity, research, and education as they applied to each clinical department. Between 1979 and 1995 the school of medicine had stopped granting tenure because of a financial downturn in the late 1970s. Dartmouth College recently concluded that it could assure the funding of 60 tenured faculty in the medical school. There are 40 individuals with tenure in the medical school at this time; tenure will be available in clinical departments at the full professor level for those who spend less than 50% time in clinical activity.

During Dr. Andrew Wallace's tenure as dean over the past 6.5 years, the school has implemented a new curriculum that has increased selective time and patient contact hours in the first 2 years. Basic science teaching relevant to clinical pharmacology and genetics has been incorporated into the teaching programs during the clinical years. Problem-based learning is spread through all 4 years of the curriculum. The dean has encouraged medical students to take expanded elective time at Dartmouth College in a variety of non-medical-related courses. Dartmouth Medical School has developed an outstanding reputation for its primary care and rural health education programs and for its work in health services research and clinical outcome studies. The school has a limited number of funded core research resources, but its research is oriented around investigator-initiated (R01) grants. There are three Ph.D. programs in the basic sciences, including cell and molecular biology, physiology, and pharmacology. There are also doctoral and masters programs in evaluative clinical sciences. The research programs in the department of psychiatry have developed within this tradition, which has also shaped the research programs at the Veterans Administration medical center at White River Junction, Vermont, an affiliated hospital.

The Department of Psychiatry at Dartmouth-Hitchcock Medical Center

Dr. Peter Silberfarb, the fourth full-time chair at Dartmouth, has held the position for the past decade. The first chair was Dr. Robert Weiss, who initially developed psychiatry as a division of internal medicine within the Hitchcock Clinic. With the establishment of the school of medicine as a 4-year school, Dr. Weiss negotiated for the creation of a department of psychiatry reporting to the dean of the medical school. Following Dr. Weiss's retirement, Dr. Peter Whybrow was recruited to Dartmouth as chair of psychiatry to help develop an academic program. Dr. Whybrow served for 6 years in this capacity and also served briefly in the dean's office. He subsequently moved on to become chair of psychiatry at the University of Pennsylvania. Dr. Whybrow was followed by Dr. Gary Tucker, who served as chair for 9 years, following his tenure as residency training director. Dr. Tucker left Dartmouth to become the chair of psychiatry at the University of Washington. When Dr. Tucker left, he was succeeded by Dr. Silberfarb.

The place of psychiatry as the only current clinical department in the school of medicine (i.e., reporting to the dean) is both a strength and a weakness.[2] The present reporting structure has enabled the department to develop some very creative public-sector linkages that would have been much more difficult to implement under the traditional model of the multispecialty group practice. However, the location of the department within the school of medicine has served to limit its input into the strategic planning for behavioral health services within the alliance directed by the hospital or within the broad venue of practice for the clinic. The Hitchcock Clinic and the Mary Hitchcock Memorial Hospital have separately been able to craft behavioral health linkages for their distinct regional strategies. The department of psychiatry, reporting to the dean of the school of medicine and linked only indirectly to the hospital and clinic, has not figured prominently in the direction of these behavioral health networks.

---

[2] Recently, the clinical activity of the department of community and family medicine joined the Hitchcock Clinic.

In the area of behavioral health services, the Lahey Clinic has a distinct department of psychiatry and behavioral medicine. The southern region of the clinic has developed a behavioral health care system under a psychologist, Dr. James Melton.[3] His program is currently operated by the clinic without the collaboration of the department of psychiatry. The department of psychiatry staffs the Community Mental Health Center in Manchester, New Hampshire (in the southern region), as part of its linkage with the public sector. Three to four years ago, 6 hospitals (including Mary Hitchcock Hospital) and 10 mental health centers created their own behavioral health network, called Blue Choice, as part of New Hampshire's Blue Cross. Mary Hitchcock Memorial Hospital is one of the owners of this behavioral health network. At least one of the affiliated mental health centers, West Central Services in Lebanon, New Hampshire, is part of the network of hospitals organized by the Mary Hitchcock Memorial Hospital. Recently, West Central Community Mental Health Center has begun to work with the department of psychiatry to create an integrated rapid assessment and triage service (see later section).

Despite the fact that the department chair reports to the dean, Dr. Silberfarb also has a vote on the board of governors of the Hitchcock Clinic (along with other clinical department heads). While there have been recent efforts to reorganize the department from the medical school to the clinic, everyone appears to recognize that the department's location has served to advance the public sector–academic linkage that would have been more difficult to implement under the clinic's structure. A rich group of state contracts also provides significant indirect cost support to the school of medicine. Because it is outside of the clinic's structure, psychiatry does its own billings and collections and managed care marketing. Apart from a deficit 6 years ago due to a shortfall in calculating bad debts and allowances, the department has remained in the black and has been able to pay back to the dean's office the funds required to bail it out of its previous deficit.

In many ways, the recent history of the department of psychiatry

---

[3] The psychiatry department was initially involved in 1989 in planning for behavioral health services in the southern region, but the effort did not succeed and the clinic created its own program under Dr. Melton.

at Dartmouth could serve as a model case study for a system undergoing change. Two years ago, Dr. Leighton Huey and Mr. David Budlong were recruited by Dr. Silberfarb from the Scripps Behavioral Health Program and the department of psychiatry at the University of California–San Diego to help the department transition to the changing health care environment. Dr. Huey and Mr. Budlong came to Dartmouth with a vision based on their experiences in the intensively managed care environment of Southern California. They have provided the vision to the department, giving feedback in relationship to the change process. They have succeeded, in part, because of the strong and consistent support they have received from the department chair. Dr. Huey serves as the vice chair for clinical programs and Mr. Budlong serves as the department administrator. Their efforts have produced cost savings of $500,000 in the past year, and they have reduced the length of stay on the inpatient units to less than 7 days. Their vision of the future brings the clinical delivery system of the department into an integrated alignment with public-sector programs and has served to make departmental programs easily accessible throughout the Dartmouth-Hitchcock Medical Center.

Mr. Budlong and Dr. Huey described their first task in preparing the department for change as faculty development. After 2 months at Dartmouth, they organized a retreat for the faculty to define the system as they found it, to define the future needs, and to describe what would need to happen for the department to succeed in the new world of health care. The most critical problem they identified involved limitations of access and clinical capacity. They have now created a group of multidisciplinary diagnostic and treatment teams consisting of faculty members, senior and junior residents, and other mental health professionals. The major focus of the teams is on ease of access for patients and referring physicians; speed of assessment, diagnosis, treatment, or referral; and a disease-management orientation. The latter focuses on functional goals, costs of care, and patient satisfaction within a system of continuous quality improvement.

The teams function within primary care practice settings—the traditional psychiatric inpatient, partial hospital, and outpatient settings—and within the specialized services (e.g., clinical neuroscience consults to neurology and neurosurgery). Dr. Harold Sox, the chair of the department of medicine, highlighted for me the change in access that he and his staff have observed in the past year. The rapid availability of solid mental health consultations in the primary care and family practice areas has changed the perception of psychiatric services among referring physicians while enhancing psychosocial and clinical services to all patients.

The new system is in place and clearly working. If it is fully successful, Dr. Huey, Dr. Silberfarb, and their colleagues will have transformed a traditional department of psychiatry into a behavioral health and psychosocial service system for the hospital and the clinic. Historical conflicts between West Central Services (the Lebanon, New Hampshire–based community mental center) and the department of psychiatry have been deemphasized in the creation of the Dartmouth-Hitchcock Behavioral Health network, which links the mental health center and the department of psychiatry in a common toll-free telephone number and triage system. Dr. Jesse Turner, the chief executive officer of the mental health center, described the evolutionary changes as profound and was optimistic that this type of initiative would lead to the development of a coherent behavioral health network throughout the broad geographic areas covered in the northern and southern strategies of the Dartmouth-Hitchcock Medical Center. Through its new staffing arrangements with the Manchester Mental Health Center, the department could be well positioned to craft this type of broad behavioral health care network.

The clinical system change has also had a profound impact on the residency training program, which has resulted in some faculty resignations. Remaining faculty appear to be increasingly enthusiastic about the linkage between their principal clinical focus and their research and academic interests. Dr. Ronald Green, the residency training director, described his work on the "brain team" with a neuropsychiatrist with a special interest in traumatic brain injury. Dr. Green spoke glowingly of the things he had learned in the context of his increased consultation activities and highlighted the heavy workload that Dr. Huey and other leaders in the department have undertaken in transforming their clinical delivery system. Dr. Huey believes that the model developed at Dartmouth could lead to a strong consortium of academic department programs organized along the same lines and operating in a tier of locations across northern New England.

Commencing in July 1995, the department implemented a Firm Model of residency training. Table 1 depicts a sample of the sequence of longitudinal and block rotation experiences over the course of the residency training program, listing the projected skills and knowledge base for graduates of the program.

In the first-year rotation on the multidisciplinary longitudinal treatment team, the residents spend 75% of their time on inpatient experiences. In the second year, the residents spend 50% time caring for

TABLE 1

Profile of the clinical psychiatrist to emerge from the training program

Knowledge base	Skills
An excellent physician and diagnostician; has core knowledge of the range of psychopathology	Can provide cost-effective, quality mental health care; will work to preserve patients' benefits, utilize benefits stringently and only as required
Skilled and knowledgeable at a mechanistic level in sophisticated psychopharmacology; strong knowledge base in drugs and drug interactions	Can interface readily with primary and tertiary care physicians and systems; can be a teacher to them and a caregiver to their patients; possesses strong consultation/liaison skills
Skilled and knowledgeable in brief therapies	Works comfortably within a multidisciplinary team system; can assume team leadership role if indicated
Has a strong knowledge of individual and group dynamics and systems	Can effectively deal with both acute and chronic patients
Has sense of economics and fiscal realities; understands implications of health care reform, managed care, and utilization management; can work quickly and efficiently	Will refer patients to the most appropriate level of care and match treatment with patient; can utilize the continuum of care in treating patients
Has the ability to comprehend research, determine quality research, and understand potential application of that research to clinical work	Has good outcomes
Has a public health perspective and population-based focus	Has demand management skills, especially for high utilizers

patients in inpatient wards. In the third year, 20%–25% of a resident's time is in inpatient settings. The block rotations at the VA and in the public sector reflect the requirements of a multisite residency training program and present something of a challenge to the longitudinal orientation (see Table 2).

All of the senior faculty with whom I spoke acknowledged the problem but were optimistic about a solution. Each multidisciplinary longitudinal treatment team includes a faculty psychiatrist, a cognitive-behaviorally oriented clinical psychologist, a case manager, a senior psychiatry resident, one or two junior residents, and a third-year medical student. Each team is responsible for a small number of patients in inpatient settings, two to three psychiatric subspecialty ambulatory care

TABLE 2

Sample sequence of longitudinal and block rotation experiences over the course of residency training at Dartmouth

PGY I

Medicine	MILTT*	
4 months	8 months	

PGY II

MILTT	Public sector	Veterans Administration
	New Hampshire Hospital	4 months (two inpatient, two
4 months	4 months	consultant)

PGY III

MILTT

PGY IV

MILTT

Half-time MILTT leader
Half-time elective

Note. Several other configurations are possible, as described in the text. For example, the PGY III or IV years can be longitudinal experiences at our VA or New Hampshire Hospital.

*MILTT are multidisciplinary longitudinal treatment teams

clinics, and backup (on a rotational basis) for two nurse practitioners who staff the psychiatry crisis service. The teams also provide specialized consultation-liaison services[4] to neurology/neurosurgery, obstetrics/gynecology, and oncology. There are also distinct rotations in primary care settings, such as the family practice center and the internal medicine clinic.

Education

The residency program has already been reduced from 36 to 26 residents. In 1995–1996, seven postgraduate year (PGY) II residents were admitted, and five PGY II residents were projected for the year 2000. The program also plans to reduce the number of child fellows from five to four but to initiate two advanced clinical fellowships and two research fellowships in the center for posttraumatic stress disorder (PTSD) and in the geriatric psychiatry program. Development of joint psychiatry family practice and joint psychiatry internal medicine residencies are expected in the next 4 years.

Dr. Ronald Green serves as director of education and training in the department of psychiatry. He is also the residency training director and has a director of medical student education (Dr. Mark Reid) reporting to him. Dr. Green rates the psychiatric residency program as the most important educational effort in the department, followed by the clerkship and the reeducation of other mental health professionals to better serve managed care. Dr. Silberfarb identified the reeducation of psychiatrists regarding managed care as the most critical educational need in the area. Primary care education was listed as the number-one priority by Dr. Huey and by Dr. Sox (the chair of medicine). If the faculty-development programs organized by Dr. Huey and his associates are included, this department will be involved heavily in the reeducation of psychiatrists and other mental health providers to better serve in the

---

[4] Because managed care accounts for a small percentage of clinical activity in the Lebanon/Hanover area, it is possible for these teams to bill on a fee-for-service basis. As the percentage of managed care and capitation increases, some of the costs of these services may have to be bundled within the charges for medical and surgical services. In the latter case, the clinic will need to develop a methodology to reimburse the department for these services.

managed care environment. Indeed, this continuing medical education activity for faculty has become a major educational initiative.[5]

The department is also involved in primary care undergraduate and graduate medical education. The chair of medicine and the leaders in the department of psychiatry agreed that the best approach to primary care education in the behavioral health area would be collaborative. Presently, the psychiatry department's educational offerings in primary care include focused case consultations, the rotation of primary care residents on psychiatry services, lectures by psychiatry faculty, and the organization of Balint groups for residents in the primary care track. Psychiatrists are involved on-site in primary care settings.

At the undergraduate medical student level, the department's clerkship has recently been extended from 7 to 8 weeks. It offers preclinical courses on the scientific basis of medicine as it relates to psychiatry (42 lecture hours, 21 seminar hours) and participates in a longitudinal clinical experience (72 lecture hours, 72 seminar hours). Elective clerkships are offered in psycho-oncology, sleep disorders, and substance abuse. The dean believes the psychiatry clerkship is one of the most successful in the school. The department is involved in further implementation of the problem-based learning curriculum, bringing clinical perspectives to teaching in neuroanatomy and other neuroscience courses.

Research

The department is the second most successful department in garnering research support at Dartmouth Medical School. The dean believes that the structure of the department within the school of medicine (versus the clinic) might have contributed to this success. One critical element has been the development of the Dartmouth–New Hampshire Psychiatric Research Center at the New Hampshire State Hospital and the West Central Mental Health Center. This program, under the direction of Dr. Robert Drake, has successfully brought in research support from the National Institute of Mental Health (NIMH) related to clinical out-

---

[5] They have not yet extended this continuing medical education effort to networked providers, but they may as they work more closely with the Lahey-Hitchcock Clinic.

comes in major mental disorders. The public-sector program at the New Hampshire State Hospital is directed by Dr. Robert Vidaver, who was recruited by Dr. Silberfarb in 1988 from the chair in psychiatry at Eastern Virginia. He, along with Dr. Silberfarb and the previous chair, Dr. Gary Tucker, laid the groundwork for the model contract wherein all 14 of the psychiatrists are Dartmouth faculty.

Three years before Dr. Vidaver's arrival, the state hospital had lost its accreditation. The hospital now is Medicaid eligible, including funds from the disproportionate share (DISH) allocations.[6] Dartmouth receives a contract from the state of New Hampshire for $3 million a year, which includes overhead support to the school of medicine. At the New Hampshire State Hospital, every admission has a full diagnostic work-up, including research rating scales. The developed model has brought several hundred thousand dollars of direct research support on chronic mental illness to the program from the state, a total that has been multiplied manyfold by support from the federal government. It has led to the creation of a model public-sector program linked to a strong academic department. Dr. Silberfarb, Dr. Huey, and Dr. Vidaver now propose to develop a statewide clinical trials program linking the programs under their direction to strengthen the clinical research opportunities within the Dartmouth and public-sector systems.

Finally, the Veterans Administration medical center at White River Junction has a strong tradition of undergraduate and graduate medical education in psychiatry, as well as a nationally known research program on PTSD. The research programs at the VA, as in the private sector, are consistent with the strong tradition of health services research in the medical school.

Summary

The department of psychiatry at Dartmouth Medical School has benefited from a strong public-sector relationship, a good working relation-

---

[6] The state of New Hampshire recently established a formal network of mental health centers under the New Hampshire State Hospital umbrella to facilitate the eligibility of outpatient mental health services for Medicaid funding.

ship with the affiliated Veterans Administration medical center, and a strong health services research program within the parent medical school. In the past 2 years, the leadership of the department has invested in a change process that could serve as a model on how to lead an integrated process of change for a clinical delivery system with substantial educational and research responsibilities. The change process has been managed with great sensitivity to the academic mission, the changing needs of the health care environment, and the human needs of faculty and staff. It has been done by bringing in effective and sensitive change agents under strong and stable leadership that was already present in the department. Although it may be difficult to replicate in other settings, the Dartmouth example should offer considerable optimism to other academic departments of psychiatry about the possibilities of change and the substantial added value that a department of psychiatry can give to the broader academic health care delivery system of the parent academic health center.

The Department of Psychiatry at the University of Maryland– Baltimore and the University of Maryland Health Sciences Center

Roger E. Meyer, M.D.

I visited the department of psychiatry at the University of Maryland Health Science Center on August 7–8, 1996. Within the health sciences center and the University of Maryland–Baltimore, I met with the dean (Donald Wilson, M.D.), the president and chief executive officer of the University of Maryland Medical System (UMMS) (Dr. Morton Rapoport), and the president of the University of Maryland–Baltimore (Dr. David Ramsay). In the department of psychiatry, I met with Dr. John Talbott (chair), Dr. George Balis (director of education and training and director of residency training), Dr. David McDuff (director of the division of managed care and the director of the division of alcohol and drug abuse), Dr. Peter Hauser (chief of psychiatry at the Baltimore Veterans Administration Medical Center), and Mr. John Regenfuss (administrator in the department of psychiatry).

Within the health sciences center, I also met with Dr. Herbert Muncie Jr., who is professor and chair of the department of family medicine. In order to assess the views of local managed behavioral health companies, I met with Dr. Henry Harbin, who is president and corporate executive officer of Green Spring Health Services. Dr. Harbin is also a psychiatrist who trained, and has been on the psychiatry faculty for many years, at the University of Maryland. Before his association with Green Spring, Dr. Harbin worked in the public sector in the state of Maryland and served as Commissioner of Mental Health in that state.

General Environment

The University of Maryland School of Medicine is the oldest medical school in Baltimore. It functions as a part of the University of Maryland–Baltimore campus, which includes a law school, pharmacy school, medical school, nursing school, graduate school, dental school, and school of social work. The campus is directed by President David Ramsay, who reports through the chancellor of the University of Maryland system campus to the board of regents. Dr. Ramsay became chancellor in 1994 and has brought vision and management skills to an already established leadership group at the medical school and in the hospital.

The hospital was privatized as a separate 501(c)3 corporation, with its own board of trustees, in 1984. Dr. Ramsay and Dean Wilson serve as members of this board of trustees. The faculty practice plan in the school of medicine was also chartered as a 501(c)3 corporation in 1987. The dean, Dr. Wilson, serves as the elected chair of the board of directors of the faculty practice plan, which functions more as a federated plan rather than a multispecialty group practice. The leadership of the campus (Dr. Ramsay), the hospital (Dr. Rapoport), and the school of medicine and faculty practice plan (Dr. Wilson and the vice chair of the board of the faculty practice plan) have come together in a planning process to deal more effectively with managed care and capitated forms of payment.

At this juncture, the hospital and practice plan have limited experience with capitation. They have developed a program of health care for university hospital employees (10,000 covered lives). The department of family medicine has capitation contracts for 7,000 covered lives, and the cardiology product line (including cardiothoracic surgery) has accepted a capitated carveout from Maryland Blue Cross and Blue Shield for 180,000 covered lives. The director of the University of Maryland Medical System (Dr. Rapoport) would like to see additional product line carveouts. (In this regard, he has been impressed with the approach being taken by Drs. David McDuff and John Talbott in psychiatry.) At this juncture, while a small number of practices in the community have been purchased by the University of Maryland Medical System, the leadership group prefers to develop a network of private practices that can be tethered together through managed care contracts, marketing, information systems, and a wide array of support services.

The hospital is currently staffed for 500 beds, with a capacity of approximately 600 beds. On the day that I visited, there were 500 patients in the hospital. As lengths of stay have declined, the hospital has been able to generate a growing number of admissions. The University of Maryland Medical System has targeted linkages and practice opportunities in West Baltimore and in areas to the west and north of the city. The regional approach differentiates the University of Maryland from Johns Hopkins, but Drs. Ramsay, Wilson, and Rapoport were unanimous in believing that there are real opportunities for collaboration between these venerable institutions. One quickly gains a sense that this leadership group prides itself in its openness and encourages discussions with any institution that would like to explore potential areas of collaboration. This attitude was borne out and validated in the separate discussions that I had with Dr. Steven Sharfstein at Sheppard-Pratt (see Sheppard-Pratt case report). Dr. Sharfstein described years of frustrated efforts to combine his residency training program with that at Johns Hopkins. He also described the responsiveness that he encountered at all levels within the University of Maryland Medical System to his proposal to merge the psychiatric residency training program at Sheppard-Pratt with that at the University of Maryland. To paraphrase Dr. Sharfstein, the University of Maryland was "content to collaborate—they didn't need to take over at Sheppard-Pratt."

In general, revenue from managed care to the hospital and the school of medicine now accounts for only 16% of the overall budget ($80 million out of $500 million). This percentage has not increased over the past 12 months. A managed care division serves the hospital and faculty practice plan within the structure of University Care. The latter is a limited liability corporation designed to protect the assets of the university, the school of medicine, and the hospital. The faculty practice plan has set up a five-member clinical practice committee that meets weekly to decide about managed care contracts. The leadership of the campus, the school, and the hospital have arranged for a number of retreats, bringing in consultants to help educate faculty on functioning in a managed care environment. One has the sense that neither the hospital nor the clinical departments are yet feeling enough financial pain from managed care to move beyond their present organizational structure.

Over the past 15 years, the University of Maryland Medical System, the University of Maryland School of Medicine, and the University of Maryland–Baltimore campus have been substantially changed by a considerable amount of new construction. While the leadership group emphasizes that their school is "not Hopkins," the research budget has been growing approximately 20% per year in the past few years and now exceeds $100 million per year. New research space has been opened, and the university recently developed a major new initiative on AIDS research that attempts to bring together public and private resources under the direction of Dr. Robert Gallo. The effort drew the strong interest and financial support of the governor's office. The productivity of the research enterprise has been further strengthened by a technology transfer office, which has generated $8.1 million in patent revenue. The program builds on the interests of the school of medicine and the law school. Law students can elect to work in this program, where they function as law clerks in a patent office. The law school and the medical school each contribute half salary to the leadership of this effort.

In the past 5 years, the school of medicine has endeavored to energize a philanthropic effort. It achieved its initial 5-year goal of $32 million within 4 years. The school is now embarked on a quiet phase of a $60 to $65 million campaign. It recognizes that it must develop general philanthropy and corporate interests. In general, the structures that have evolved in the school of medicine, in the clinical delivery system, and in the organization and development of research have brought together the public resources of a state university and the reasonably unfettered entrepreneurial energies of freestanding nonprofit corporations.

In the past few years, the educational programs for medical students have undergone significant change. A problem-based learning curriculum has been implemented for all 4 years of the curriculum. It is of interest that oversight for this program is chaired by a faculty member in psychiatry. There is now a required clerkship in family medicine, along with efforts to increase ambulatory care education and continuity of family care in the curriculum. Options for more research time for motivated students have been developed in the context of a research track. Both President Ramsay and Dean Wilson emphasized the importance of teaching patient care in the context of cultural sensitivity. The latter will require some effort at faculty development, and such efforts will also be important if medical students are to more effectively learn the business aspects of health care, informatics, and the delivery of clinical services in multidisciplinary teams. While graduate medical education is primarily a hospital-based function, the medical school has an office of graduate medial education (GME) that arranges institutional reviews of residency training programs on a regular cycle to help departments anticipate the regular residency review committee (RRC) reviews of their training programs.

The Department of Psychiatry at the University of Maryland

Dr. John Talbott has been chair of the department of psychiatry at the University of Maryland for the past 11 years. He is the fourth full-time chair at Maryland. The first incumbent was recruited in the 1950s. Prior to Dr. Talbott's recruitment, the department of psychiatry at Maryland had a strong tradition of public sector–academic department collaboration around a model of residency training in the public sector called the Maryland Plan. There is a strong tradition of University of Maryland residency graduates entering the public sector to serve in state hospital systems throughout Maryland. A state hospital and community mental health center was constructed on the University of Maryland–Baltimore campus in the 1970s. At the present time, trainees rotate through this facility and university faculty staff the doctoral-level positions. Dr. Talbott's long-standing commitment to public sector–academic relationships has served to strengthen the department's commitment to the public sector.

The department of psychiatry is organized into distinct functional-, content-, and institutionally based units for representation within an executive committee structure. Distinct and substantive divisions are responsible for clinical care and education within distinct subspecialties such as alcohol and drug abuse, child and adolescent psychiatry, community psychiatry, consultation-liaison psychiatry, geriatric psychiatry, and clinical psychology. The two major centers of research (the Maryland Psychiatric Research Center and the Center for Mental Health Services Research) are represented on the executive committee in the context of research. The educational program is represented and includes oversight for medical student education, residency and fellowship training, the psychology internship, and continuing medical education. The public sector is represented in this forum as the lead agency, with distinct community-based responsibilities. The adult and child clinical programs within the medical center are represented with oversight for the clinical services in addiction; consultation-liaison psychiatry; inpatient, outpatient, and day hospital employee assistance programs (EAPs); and other areas of faculty practice. Finally, the leadership of the Carter Mental Health Center (CMHC) (the state hospital/CMHC on campus), and the leadership of the psychiatric service at the Veterans Administration medical center in Baltimore, are also represented. It appears that the departmental organizational structure is matrixlike.

Commencing on July 1, 1996, the department established a division on managed behavioral health headed by Dr. David McDuff, who is also serving as director of the division on alcohol and drug abuse. While professional fee billings account for only 5% of the department's budget, it has established the division on managed care to better align the present and future practice activities of the department with the overall plans of the University of Maryland Medical System. Through linkages in the department, efforts are being made to better integrate activities in the public sector with those in the University of Maryland Medical System. The department is anticipating the day when the state may choose to privatize the Medicaid program.

Finally, the department has learned a great deal about the linkage between EAP and managed behavioral health through its management of the EAP system for the medical center. Indeed, the new managed care division is utilizing the leadership of the EAP to coordinate managed behavioral health contracting for the department, in conjunction with medical center–wide efforts. Dr. Talbott and the new division director for managed care, Dr. McDuff, reported that, between 1993 and 1996, the length of stay on the adult inpatient units in the hospital have declined from 19 to 8 days. The census has been maintained by a near doubling of admissions per year. The length of stay on the child psychiatry inpatient unit has been more resistant to change. In addition to the reduced length of stay, the department has been able to establish four day hospitals, an ultrashort stay unit, and 24-hour-a-day availability for urgent care. One of the goals of the new division is to establish a network of university-associated clinicians in the community. The department has been successful in placing its mental health professionals within the primary care practice settings of the medical center and the department of family medicine. The department also has a well-regarded inpatient medical psychiatric consultation program, as well as a wide-ranging inpatient and outpatient addiction consultation service.

In relationship to the faculty practice plan for psychiatry, Dr. Talbott made the following points: The information systems platform does not work for psychiatry because it is geared to the needs of high-volume practitioners and highly specialized tertiary care. The department does not use the appointment structure in the faculty practice plan and is taxed excessively for the costs of malpractice. There are no discipline-specific standards of productivity, and there are huge inefficiencies in billings and collections. At the present time, more than 58% of total charges in the department of psychiatry are bad debts and allowances. There is a flat dean's tax of 11.2% for all collections.

Within the faculty practice, each physician is designated with a separate account from which charges for malpractice and other services are withdrawn. In the department of psychiatry, there are apparently 39 such accounts. Although the department pays an inclusive fee for billings and collections and managed care marketing, the department is not charged for space, medical records, or physician extenders. There is a 7% charge to support the administrative costs of the practice plan. Given the patient mix (with the high rate of bad debts and allowances) and the inefficiencies and charges of the practice, it is no wonder that the public-sector relationships have become so important to the present and future of this department. Given the history, the new division of managed care will need to move vigorously to create a community-based network of clinicians if it is to work effectively with managed behavioral health companies and if the department hopes to secure managed care activity within the medical center.

During the 11 years of Dr. Talbott's tenure, the department has never been in deficit. The department's budget consists of a blend of funds from the university, the state of Maryland, community service contracts, hospital administrative income, state-based training funds, and federal research support. In fiscal year 1995, the department reported a surplus of more than $800,000. In this context, morale in the department appeared to be excellent, with real optimism regarding the possibilities for fulfilling individual goals and the department's mission.

Educational Programs

The department is responsible for a broad array of educational programs, including 14 lecture hours and 14 seminar hours in the behavioral and social sciences, 20 lecture hours and 20 seminar hours on psychopathology (including psychopharmacology), and 1 hour of lecture and 10 hours of seminar on psychiatric interviewing. The department participates in the introduction to clinical medicine with 30 hours contributed per year by full-time faculty and 20 hours per year contributed by voluntary faculty. Until this year, the department supported a 6-week clerkship, which has been reduced to 4 weeks in the context of the reorganization of the curriculum. The chair of the committee overseeing problem-based learning in the medical school is a psychiatrist, Dr. David Mallott, who was also a past Teacher of the Year Award recipient. Four-week clinical electives are offered on eating disorders, consultation psychiatry, and community psychiatry. Until recently, the percentage of medical school graduates of the University of Maryland entering psychiatry equaled or exceeded national percentages. In 1995 and 1996, the percentage dropped below the national average. Similarly, in recent years the Maryland residency has relied on international medical graduates to fill out its class.

Commencing in 1997, the psychiatric residency program at the University of Maryland will be merged with its counterpart at Sheppard-Pratt. In the old configuration, Sheppard-Pratt had 30 residency slots and the University of Maryland 60. In the new configuration, Sheppard-Pratt will be paying for 20 slots and the university will be paying for 54 slots. When fully operational, the merged program will represent a 17% decrease in the number of graduates compared with a time when the programs were independent. In addition to the residency slots, the department offers advanced clinical fellowships in geriatric psychiatry (four slots), addiction psychiatry (two slots), forensic psychiatry (two slots), research (two slots), and consultation-liaison psychiatry (two slots). No decreases are projected in these numbers. Dr. Talbott projects increasing the number of research fellowships to four by the year 2000. For the future, Dr. Talbott projects more longitudinal experiences for residents in integrated settings and more training in ambulatory care and primary care settings.

As projected, the merged training program would appear to be a fairly traditional multisite experience involving the University of Maryland, the Veterans Administration, Sheppard-Pratt, and specialty rotations on child psychiatry, consultation psychiatry, and addiction psychiatry. Dr. George Balis, director of education, is a strong advocate of traditional values in psychiatric education. He regards the five most critical skills for psychiatrists for the future to include long-term psychotherapy, treating very sick people well, the art of psychopharmacology, working in systems in leadership roles, and developing alternatives to managed behavioral health. Some of the educational leadership in the department have strong negative views about the impact of managed care on psychiatry.

Dr. Talbott listed the five most critical skills as being the provision of cost effective and efficient care with a short-term focus, effective assessment and triage, the ability to perform self monitoring to work in capitated settings, the maintenance of a science-based practice, and the development of skills for the future including telemedicine and informatics within psychiatric practice. He believes strongly that the educational programs need to reach out to clinicians in practice as part of the effort to create quality assurance within a network of affiliated clinicians. Dr. Henry Harbin, the chief executive officer of Green Springs, listed diagnostic and treatment planning, the management of high-risk patients, the cost-effective use of inpatient care, the management of less severe patients in multidisciplinary teams, and the integration of pharmacological and psychosocial intervention as the most important skills for psychiatrists. The conflict between traditional views of psychiatric practice and managed behavioral health would appear to be playing out within the department rather than between the department and the managed care sector.

In addition to the department's role in the education of medical students and psychiatric residents, it presently offers training for 4 psychology interns, 5 social work students, 10 masters-prepared nurses, 12 baccalaureate nurses, and 12 occupational therapists per year. Dr. Talbott projects an increase in the number of social work students being trained (from 5 to 10) and of occupational therapy students (from 12 to 16) by the year 2000. The department also participates in the education of primary care physicians. Psychiatry faculty provide focused case consultation in primary care settings, some primary care residents rotate on psychiatry, psychiatry faculty offer lectures and seminars to primary care residents, and Balint groups are offered to primary care residents and faculty in the department of family medicine. The principal psychiatrists involved in the primary care site education are addiction psychiatrists; the consultation-liaison psychiatry faculty and fellows tend to focus on the inpatient setting.

The chair of family medicine, Dr. Herbert Muncie, spoke very positively about the growing role of psychiatrists in his family medicine education programs over the past 2 to 4 years. A current resident in family medicine spends half of his or her time in the addiction fellowship. Dr. Muncie believes that the residency programs in family medicine will increasingly require knowledge of psychosocial aspects of patient care and that family practice physicians and other primary care clinicians need to learn how to manage their time and their lives. In all of this, he saw an important role for psychiatry in the education programs of family medicine and primary care physicians. Dr. Muncie believes that primary care physicians should be familiar with the types of diagnoses and emotional problems encountered in primary care settings, the principles of treatment for these disorders and problems, and when to refer or to ask for psychiatric consultation. Although he believes that primary care physicians could provide primary care services to the severely mentally ill, he does not think that these physicians should be trained to use more complex pharmacological agents such as neuroleptic and mood-stabilizing drugs.

Research Programs

The research programs of the department of psychiatry at Maryland have three major strengths: schizophrenia research at the Maryland Psychiatric Research Center headed by Dr. William Carpenter (staffed by faculty from the University of Maryland and funded by the Maryland Department of Mental Hygiene), health services research at the university, and a new neuroendocrine-based research program at the Veterans Administration medical center in Baltimore. The program in health services research has been strongly encouraged by Dr. Talbott and is now one of the strongest health services research programs among psychiatry departments in the United States. All of the department's research programs appear to be vital and vibrant. The potential weak link in the research portfolio is the line item placement of the Maryland Psychiatric Research Center in the state budget and the growing turbulence consequent to changes in the Veterans Administration medical center. With regard to the latter, positions in psychiatry have been frozen as the regional network is being formed. In the past year, the department at the VA hospital has lost four full-time psychiatrists and a number of nursing positions. Important units in substance abuse and PTSD are being closed. The university will have to make a major effort within the new structure to assure continued commitment by the Veterans Administration to the academic collaboration. University leadership has been extremely active in the past when the line item budget for the Maryland Psychiatric Research Center was threatened in the appropriations process of the state legislature. An awareness of the importance of this program to the university was communicated to me at the highest levels.

The department of psychiatry has managed to develop strong research resources of its own and effective collaborations in brain imaging (positron-emission tomography [PET]), genetics, epidemiology, and functional magnetic resonance imaging (MRI). Surprisingly, the medical center does not have a general clinical research center (GCRC) from the National Institutes of Health (NIH). However, the medical center has a small grants program and directly funds departments to facilitate new research initiatives. In general, the research programs of the department and the medical center continue to be in a growth phase and seem able to combine public and private resources in creative ways.

Summary

The department of psychiatry at the University of Maryland has benefited from a strong public-sector relationship; good to excellent relationships among the Baltimore campus of the University of Maryland, the school of medicine, and the hospital; and an ability to blend public- and private-sector initiatives. Dr. Talbott has been an active leader as chair and is now attempting to confront the challenges of managed behavioral health. While the department's budget is not at risk from managed care, the future of its public-sector program could depend on the department's ability to craft an effective integrated network. The newly merged residency education program with Sheppard-Pratt presents a significant challenge—and opportunity—to the department and Sheppard-Pratt to develop an educational program consistent with the demands of the new clinical environment.

The Sheppard and Enoch Pratt Hospital, Towson, Maryland

Roger E. Meyer, M.D

I visited the Sheppard and Enoch Pratt Hospital on Friday, February 17, 1996, and met with the president and chief executive officer, Dr. Steven Sharfstein and Dr. Robert Schreter. Dr. Schreter is the medical director of the hospital's health plan and also participates in the consultation service of the American Psychiatric Association.

General Environment

I had been eager to meet with Dr. Sharfstein following discussions that we had at a meeting of the editorial board of the *American Journal of Psychiatry,* where he told me that his residency training program was about to be merged with the residency training program at the University of Maryland. The motivation for the merger was to cut costs of education in a hospital that has the second largest endowment of any private psychiatric hospital ($63 million–$3 million per year of income). The institution has also gone furthest in meeting the challenge of managed care. Nevertheless, because the institution was losing (by its estimate) $1 million per year in its training programs, it elected to merge these programs with those of the University of Maryland. If this institution, which has crafted one of the most sophisticated approaches to managed care and a partnering with the public sector, is unable to support clinical education from "surplus" clinical dollars, the situation must be instructive for academic departments of psychiatry.

Dr. Sharfstein was quite explicit with me: "The primary mission of Sheppard Pratt is services." On the hierarchy of values, a learning environment is not the defining principle, although the institution has a long tradition of viewing psychiatric education as a priority, using patients as part of the teaching process. This tradition has continued even though lengths of stay now average 5 days. The $3 million per year income from the institution's endowment was, by the terms of the original bequest, to be charity care, especially for Quakers. The system has now evolved to the point where fully 75% of patients within the system are patients supported by public dollars.

Sheppard-Pratt directs three community mental health centers covering a population of 600,000 to 700,000 individuals. Its 322 beds have now been pared to 180 (and soon to 150 beds); the institution is running an average daily census of 140 patients. It has 12 day programs, 2 of which have been incorporated on the inpatient units and run 7 days per week, as well as 10 off-unit partial hospital programs (PHPs), with four of these off grounds. Lengths of stay in the partial hospital programs are running 30 days or less, even for patients with chronic schizophrenia. Sheppard-Pratt has developed partial hospital programs as specialized clinical programs (e.g., chemical dependency, eating disorders, and child psychiatry).

The institution has had to reinvent the business. It views its core business as behavioral health care and not hospital care. To survive financially, it has had to accept capitated risk-based contracts. Parenthetically, the largest contract is a subcapitated contract with Kaiser. Under this contract Sheppard-Pratt has received $3 to $4 per member per month (PMPM), including the costs of inpatient care, on a capitated basis. Kaiser wishes to negotiate this sum downward, and Sheppard-Pratt will be demanding that more of the care be offered by primary care physicians at Kaiser. Before signing its Kaiser contract, the institution secured actuarial assistance but has commented that the problem with capitated contracts (or subcapitated contracts) is not only getting actuarial advice but also securing accurate data.

In order to survive financially, Sheppard-Pratt has had to develop direct contracts for employee assistance programs (EAPs), which now cover a number of businesses and 150,000 lives at the *Washington Post*, local banks, law firms, and so forth. The EAPs offer six visits and referral. The institution has other nationwide contracts for which it receives $8 to $10 PMPM, covering approximately 15,000 people. It offers a discounted fee-for-services rate to local providers (outside the area) on these national contracts. The behavioral health carveouts offer less of an opportunity for integrated care than the contract that Sheppard-Pratt has with Kaiser. It also serves as the third-party administrator for Alex Brown (the investment firm), where it is completely at risk. Additionally, the institution has developed the capacity to provide administrative management services.

Sheppard-Pratt serves a large number of patients in the public sector in Baltimore County and Hartford County. It runs three community mental health centers (CMHCs) under contract with the county using state dollars. The contract includes special programs such as geriatric home treatment. Under the terms of the contracts, all of the CMHC employees are employees of Sheppard-Pratt. When Medicaid becomes "managed" in Maryland, Sheppard-Pratt expects to compete for the business with other community mental health centers and may join with managed care companies in order to keep its present business. If the entire state is carved out in terms of behavioral health services, Sheppard-Pratt is prepared to be involved in a joint venture. Present contracts with the public sector are for 3 years and can be renegotiated on an annual basis. State dollars are also available for the treatment of persons with chemical dependency. Sheppard-Pratt has developed an on-grounds residential treatment center for chemical dependency, with a length of stay of 11 days, and medical detoxification at the nearby Greater Baltimore Medical Center. With the exception of the chemical dependence program (directed by a psychologist), all service lines are run by psychiatrists.

Sheppard-Pratt has had a practice plan for a number of years that rewards productivity. In the past 3 years (the length of time of the practice plan), staff have been seeing 30% more patients with 20% fewer psychiatrists. Last year the system gave out $800,000 in bonuses. The greatest single innovation that enabled the institution to move in this direction was the introduction of an expensive information system.

Details of the merged residency training program are offered in the case report from the University of Maryland. Sheppard-Pratt expects to save money in this merger of training programs. It will decrease the total number of residents in both programs. A comparable reduction in faculty numbers and in space at Sheppard-Pratt will also be necessary. The present program costs $1 million per year to run. By the year 2000 the institution expects that the cost will be $500,000 per year instead of an earlier-projected $1.4 million per year.

The Department of Psychiatry at Stanford University

Roger E. Meyer, M.D.

I visited the department of psychiatry at Stanford University School of Medicine on February 21–22, 1996. I had meetings with Dr. Alan Schatzberg (chair of the department of psychiatry), Eugene Bauer (dean), Mr. Peter Van Etten (chief executive officer of the Stanford Health System), Dr. Peter Gregory (chief medical officer of the Stanford Health System), Dr. Barr Taylor (director of psychiatric residency training), Dr. Richard Maaze (chief of staff at the Palo Alto Veterans Administration [VA] Hospital), Dr. Michael Jacobs (head of the primary care section in general internal medicine), and Ms. Barbara Keller (executive director of the Mid-Peninsula Health Group). I also had a telephone conversation with Dr. William Goldman, vice president for medical affairs at U.S. Behavioral Health Corporation, which provides behavioral carveout programs in Northern California.

General Environment

The Stanford University School of Medicine is a relatively small medical school with a strong commitment to research excellence and productivity. The emphasis on research, with strong basic science programs and a strong emphasis on research productivity in reviewing faculty for promotion in all departments, grew with the relocation of the medical school from its former clinical site in San Francisco to the Stanford University campus in the late 1950s. When the medical school was relocated, a new hospital was constructed as part of the medical center complex. Stanford University Hospital relies significantly on admissions from community-based physicians and surgeons, especially those in nearby group practices such as the Palo Alto Clinic. Thus, from the 1950s until recently, the interests of the hospital were not fully aligned with the interests of the faculty practice plan. The hospital had a distinct governing structure from the medical school, even as it was owned by Stanford University.

In the early 1990s, following a gift of the Packard family, a consolidated children's hospital was constructed adjacent to the Stanford University Hospital, with connections at every floor. The children's hospital is separately managed and governed.[1] The faculty practice in the department of pediatrics is separately managed from the rest of the faculty practice plan, although the chair of the department of pediatrics is represented ex officio within the new practice organization at the Stanford University Medical Center.

With the arrival of a new university president in 1992, and the growing impact of managed care on academic medical centers throughout California, the board of trustees at Stanford University initiated a reexamination of the structure of the clinical delivery systems under Stanford's ownership. Thus was born a new corporate entity, the Stanford Health System (SHS), which has a distinct board of trustees with substantial corporate expertise. The initial intent of the system was to bring together the resources of Stanford University Hospital, the full-time faculty practice plan (FPP), affiliated faculty, and local group practices. Between 1993 and 1995 the leadership of the hospital (Mr. Kenneth Bloehm) and the faculty practice plan (Mr. Donald Tower), as well as the dean/vice president of the school of medicine (Dr. David Korn) resigned from their positions. The chief financial officer of the university,

---

[1] The children's hospital has recently (September 1996) been merged with Stanford Health Services, but it had previously been separately managed and governed.

Mr. Peter Van Etten, was named the chief executive officer of the Stanford Health System. Dr. Eugene Bauer (formerly chair of dermatology) was named dean of the school of medicine.

Initial efforts to bring together the full-time and affiliated physicians proved to be a failure. The full-time faculty were then organized into the Stanford faculty practice group, which established a seemingly traditional governing structure. The practice committee, which meets biweekly, is chaired by the chief medical officer of the Stanford Health System, Dr. Peter Gregory. There are 14 service-based seats on this committee; in reality the group consists of 10 department chairs and 5 nonchairs. The six clinical department chairs who are not represented are invited to all meetings but do not vote. Voting positions of the chairs are held for up to 3 years. There are three elected members (one each from hospital-, medical-, and surgical-based departments), each elected for 2 years; they may serve for up to three terms. Dr. Gregory's response to how the old system had been improved upon was that the new system is more conducive to decision making, partially because of a good contracts committee that is able to quickly decide on managed care contracts.

The new system, as did the old, places the responsibility for budget balancing at the department level. There is no sharing of profits. The dean, the SHS chief executive officer, and the chief medical officer all indicated that for the first 3 months of the fiscal year (starting September 1995), three of the five core clinical departments (surgery, obstetrics/gynecology, and psychiatry) were in deficit. The apparent deficit in the SHS account for psychiatry has resulted in the reduction of secretarial support for all psychiatry faculty and the virtual elimination of departmental support for subscriptions, dues, and travel. Moreover, faculty did not get raises until the end of the first quarter of this fiscal year because of the apparent deficit in the department. There is a 7% dean's tax based on total revenue (the same as for the department of surgery). The department believes that 7% is the lowest tax rate in the school. In the department of psychiatry, the deficit is almost exactly equal to the allocated indirect costs imposed by SHS on practice activity.

The quality of services offered by SHS to departments is unclear. In the case of the department of psychiatry, it has hired the executive director of the Mid-Peninsula Health Group for up to 2 days per week to market the department's managed care activity. The department has contracted with this group to manage its behavioral health care capitation pool and to provide a central intake structure. Under the capitation arrangement, the department's specialized services are offered on a discounted fee-for-service basis that is relatively favorable for medication management, assessment, and complex care. The fact that this marketing arrangement is paid for as a direct cost to the department, and was unknown to Dr. Gregory, suggests that there is a substantial detachment between the needs of the clinical departments (certainly psychiatry) and the services offered by the structure of SHS.

Strategic planning for SHS resides within the five-person executive group including the chief executive officer, chief financial officer, chief medical officer, chief operating officer, and chief of marketing and sales. SHS is governed by a board of 15 individuals, including the dean, the SHS chief executive officer, one department chair, the chief medical officer, one university trustee, the president of the university, and eight outside directors. The board has constituted a number of committees, including an audit committee, a compensation committee (to review the compensation of the chief executive officer), a finance committee, and a program review committee. Although Mr. Van Etten emphasized that the creation of SHS did not constitute a takeover of the medical school by the hospital, departments now receive their clinical income through SHS. Under the old faculty practice, revenue flowed directly from practice activity into the departments, and the faculty practice plan reported to the school of medicine.

Despite serious efforts to make clinical activities at Stanford more efficient and competitive, the present structure places considerable responsibility for financial performance at the level of clinical departments. The latter lack adequate information about (and control of) central administrative costs allocated to them, which account for significant expenses. If a department is in a deficit situation, it is asked to make a presentation to the finance committee of SHS. Unfortunately, there are still many operational problems in the new system that complicate the problems at the departmental level. In responding to questions raised about the department's fiscal year 1996 budget, Dr. Schatzberg identified substantial errors and oversights by SHS that resulted in a failure to bill adequately for sleep disorder assessments. If corrected, the department might actually have recorded a surplus.

The Stanford faculty practice group has clearly not evolved into a multispecialty practice plan. Its members are debating a potential evolution into a multispecialty practice plan using related value units (RVUs) to calculate the distribution of revenue dollars—particularly from any capitation. Mr. Van Etten (the SHS chief executive officer) expects that the net effect of this plan would be the transfer of some dollars from the surgical specialties to the departments of internal medicine and obstetrics. Mr. Van Etten is not convinced that the multispecialty practice model is necessarily the best route to go. He believes that this model was unsuccessful for the Sharp Health System in Southern California, but that product line service carveouts for heart disease, cancer, radiology, and behavioral health may be a more viable and realistic strategy. The present system has been very disadvantageous to psychiatry, which might be better served in a decentralized system.

Under the previous hospital chief executive officer, Mr. Bloehm, Stanford acquired several local primary care group practices. This strategy apparently continued into the early days of SHS. Indeed, while there is no department of family medicine at Stanford, the family physicians formerly employed by the Mid-Peninsula Health Group were brought into the primary care practice space adjacent to the full-time faculty in the division of internal medicine section on primary care practice under Dr. Michael Jacobs. Curiously, while these physicians now practice in the same environment, they do not appear to be incorporated into a single primary care practice. Indeed, Dr. Jacobs expressed serious concern about the intentions of SHS regarding the future of primary care. His concerns were certainly validated in my discussions with Mr. Van Etten, who pointed out that SHS was losing a great deal of money on the practices that it had purchased and in its own primary care practice. Rather than develop a network of primary care physicians, Stanford will now attempt to position itself as the tertiary care provider of choice to managed care organizations and primary care practices in the community.

SHS is presently involved in discussions with Kaiser about potential clinical collaboration. If these discussions prove fruitful, Kaiser would use the Stanford University Hospital for its tertiary care hospital needs in Northern California. The proposed arrangement would replace the primary care initiative and also enable Kaiser physicians to admit directly to Stanford University Hospital. This could produce potential conflict between specialists within the Permanente Group and the full-time Stanford faculty (and other affiliated faculty and groups, such as the Palo Alto Clinic). These issues will need to be addressed because the hospital must retain the loyalty of the Palo Alto Clinic and others. Because Kaiser of Northern California is moving to strengthen psychiatric services to its members, the change in providers could represent a significant opportunity for Stanford's department of psychiatry, if it can move quickly to effect a local delivery network. SHS has not begun to think about this opportunity.

At the time of my visit, Stanford University Medical Center and the University of California–San Francisco (UCSF) had already begun discussions that could result in the merger of some clinical programs. The recent decision by Stanford and UCSF to align their clinical delivery systems could be critical to Stanford in its proposed relationship with Kaiser because Stanford's plans to serve as the tertiary care provider for a number of health maintenance organizations (HMOs) might be jeopardized by a linkage with Kaiser. A link to UCSF could create a tertiary care system with broad geographic penetration in Northern California.

The movement away from primary care was reflected in conversations with the dean, the leadership of SHS (Mr. Van Etten and Dr. Gregory), and the head of the section on primary care (Stanford Medical Group). Not counting VA faculty, there are only nine primary care internists at Stanford and no primary care residency, although there is a family practice residency based in San Jose (Stanford affiliated). General internal medicine includes preventive medicine (Jack Farquhar), informatics, education, and the practice. Each clinician has a panel of 2,000 patients, a number that can be reduced by 10% for teaching. The primary care physicians feel the absence of a group practice mentality at Stanford. Although 60% of the primary care practice is related to HMOs, specialized surgical programs are still overwhelmingly fee-for-service systems from outside referrals.

The primary care internists welcome the presence of a psychiatric resident in the practice area, but there has been little contact between the head of the Stanford Medical Group and the head of consultation-liaison psychiatry to jointly plan a relevant program. The primary care internists expressed an interest in learning more from psychiatry on topics like domestic violence, sexual inadequacy, attention-deficit hyperactivity disorder (ADHD) in adults, borderline personality disorder, and more about new approaches to the treatment of anxiety disorders. But the future of the primary care treatment programs leaves doubts about the long term. The primary care physicians complain that there is no infrastructure support of the managed care practice for them, no adequate information system, and no resources to operate efficiently in a managed care primary care setting. The same issues apply to the place of psychiatry in SHS.

Until recently, the separate governance of children's services also made comprehensive planning for primary care (general pediatrics) and psychiatry (child/adolescent psychiatry) extremely difficult. The recruitment of a new head of child psychiatry rested with the chief executive officer of the children's hospital and the chair of pediatrics, since they controlled the resources that were to be directed to this clinical, educational, and research program.

The Department of Psychiatry at Stanford

Dr. Alan Schatzberg became chair of the department of psychiatry in 1991 following a long vacancy after the retirement and death of the previous incumbent. Dr. Schatzberg had a distinguished prior career as a clinical investigator on affective disorders and as an expert clinician and senior hospital administrator at McLean Hospital and the Massachusetts Mental Health Center. He describes the primary mission of his department "to make fundamental discoveries which expand the understanding of the causes and treatments for psychiatric disorders . . . and to facilitate the movement from fundamental discoveries to diagnosis and treatment of disease. In order to accomplish this mission, the department maintains a vigorous and diverse set of research programs in both clinical and basic science disciplines." He also highlights the department's commitment to fellowship training and residency education, along with the education of medical students.

The department's budget and programs certainly conform to the

vision that Dr. Schatzberg communicated. Research and research training support accounted for 61% of departmental income in fiscal year
1995. Gifts and endowment (also related to research) accounted for
another 14% of departmental income, while clinical revenues accounted
for only 17% of the departmental budget. Dr. Schatzberg noted that
academic departments at Stanford with substantial research support "still
have some leverage with the school," but the high practice overhead
produced an apparent deficit in the SHS budget for psychiatry (a relatively minor part of the department's budget), drawing a great deal of
negative attention in the new environment. Moreover, the department
needs to recruit for a number of endowed professorships to replace
faculty who have died, retired, or moved to other schools. One of the
most productive programs, the sleep disorders program, is uniquely tied
to a senior member of the faculty. Consequently, it is clear that if the
department is to maintain its edge in research, it will need to be freed
from the high costs of its clinical programs and the university will need
to identify ways to foster recruitment of new faculty. This issue will be
critical to the future of this department.

Clinical Activities

With the recruitment of the current chair, efforts were made to increase
the department's involvement in clinical activities. The hospital reconfigured inpatient space for two units, and a new building was constructed
for outpatient, partial hospital program (PHP), clinical research, and
educational purposes. Mr. Van Etten (the SHS chief executive officer)
believes that while the inpatient unit is generally doing well, the unit
will be relocated if the Kaiser deal goes through. The department and
the hospital seem to have no disagreement about the viability of a change
in location. The real problem is related to the overhead costs in the
outpatient area. Financial losses in the alcohol and drug program could
result in downsizing or elimination of this program. The department
and SHS are investigating the potential benefits of having both the alcohol
and drug treatment program and the sleep disorders clinic reorganized
as outpatient hospital programs. The hospital would assume—and re-
coup—costs for institutional and technical components, while the department would bill the professional components for these services. The

sleep disorders program provides referrals to private ears, nose, and throat surgeons on the Stanford faculty who operate on patients with sleep apnea, and a Stanford sleep disorders clinic has been established in San Francisco.

Many of the issues affecting the department's clinical operations within the structure of SHS have been described previously. The complexities of managed care in the rapidly changing and highly competitive behavioral health industry cannot be overestimated. The department's approach to managed care is built around an alliance with Mid Peninsula Health Center, a group practice of mental health professionals recently purchased by a for-profit corporation, Apogee. The arrangement has met some of the needs of the department, but it has stood in the way of a potential linkage with U.S. Behavioral Health (USBH) Corporation (and perhaps other managed behavioral health companies). USBH does not want to deal with Stanford through Mid Peninsula (according to Dr. William Goldman of USBH). USBH has worked out a very favorable discounted fee-for-service arrangement with the psychiatry department at UCSF (according to that institution's department chair) and would have liked the same arrangement with Stanford—"but Stanford's faculty are not really ready or interested in managed care," according to Goldman and Barbara Keller, of Mid Peninsula Health Center. The arrangement with Mid Peninsula was viewed very favorably by Ms. Keller and by the department administrator, Ms. Jane De Young. Indeed, it seems likely that without the arrangement with Mid Peninsula, Stanford's outpatient programs would not have much (if any) managed care activity, and there would be no good way for the department to take on risk-based capitation.

As described earlier, the family physicians of Mid-Peninsula Health Center were bought out by Stanford and moved to its primary care practice site, leaving the mental health professionals behind in the old program. The latter formed a group practice and developed contracts for behavioral health services. With the arrival of Alan Schatzberg, a clinical link was formed between Stanford's psychiatry program and Mid-Peninsula. The department (under Dr. Schatzberg's leadership) altered its approach to clinical service, opening a medical/psychiatry unit, as well as a separate locked unit in the hospital. The department established a variety of PHP programs, but the bed charges at Stanford University Hospital are too high for managed behavioral health services.

Mid-Peninsula Health Center offers itself as an intake and referral service to Stanford's specialty outpatient psychiatry clinics and has also provided some education on managed care to faculty in the department. Mid-Peninsula accepts risk under capitation and pays SHS for psychiatric services on a discounted fee-for-service basis. Some contracts pay only $0.75 per member per month (PMPM) for outpatient mental health services; better programs pay $1.50 PMPM. The capitation does not include the costs of hospital care (or PHP). The professional fee component of these efforts is at a case rate, which is set high. The discounted fee-for-service rates that Stanford receives favor evaluations and pharmacotherapy management. The rate for psychotherapy is the same for all licensed providers in the pool, $65 per hour.

Mid-Peninsula has also served as a bridge between Stanford Medical Group (the primary care practice) and the department of psychiatry. Mid-Peninsula receives a capitated subcontract for the 25,000 covered lives in this program. Efforts are made to direct these patients to Stanford psychiatry. Mid-Peninsula and Stanford psychiatry staff also provide joint utilization review (UR). It is certainly of interest that Barbara Keller (of Mid Peninsula) and the managed care director of UCSF psychiatry are now in discussion about connecting their activities. This issue did not come up in my discussions with the chair at UCSF, with Alan Schatzberg, or with Bill Goldman of USBH.

Educational Programs

The department of psychiatry is responsible for 12 hours of lectures (and 15 hours of clinical seminars) in the first-year medical student curriculum on psychological medicine and 18 hours of lectures (and 9 clinical seminar hours) in the second-year course on psychopathology. The required psychiatric clerkship is 4 weeks' duration. Preclinical education did not rank highly as a priority for the dean or the department. The department will be challenged to craft a meaningful clerkship that places greater emphasis on ambulatory teaching in the context of a 4-week clerkship.

The dean of the Stanford Medical School, Dr. Gene Bauer, has been in his position for approximately 1 year, following the resignation of the longtime dean and vice president, Dr. David Korn. Dr. Bauer listed his priorities for the educational activities of the psychiatry department starting with residency education, clerkship education, introduction to clinical medicine, the reeducation of psychiatrists in practice, the re-education of other mental health professionals, and preclinical courses, in that order. He listed primary care education last. He noted that this order really conforms to Stanford's vision of itself: "Stanford is about excellence which is founded on discipline-based research." This philosophy, which does not endorse primary care in a major way, was reinforced during a faculty retreat.

Dr. Bauer presented me with his vision of medical student education, consisting of a core of concentric circles. The innermost core relates to primary care disciplines, including general internal medicine, pediatrics, and obstetrics. In the next core are psychiatry, dermatology, ophthalmology, orthopedics, and gynecology. He believes that the future of the graduate medical education system is in ambulatory and primary care, with a number of disciplines contributing to primary care education. He notes that there will be a downsizing of some specialist providers. The proposed linkage with the University of California–San Francisco is already focused on some of these cooperative areas, including neurosurgery, dermatology, and anesthesiology. He emphasized the importance of psychiatry in other areas of medical practice as well, noting that the department of psychiatry is a successful research department and that more income comes from research than from clinical services.

Dean Bauer shared the strategic planning document summary with me:

Thirty-five years ago the University Trustees decided to move the medical school from San Francisco to Palo Alto, their goals were . . . to transform the medical school into a world class center for biomedical research, education and clinical care. . . . Our challenge is to refocus and reconfigure ourselves in a way that will preserve our core academic functions and provide a measure of financial stability. . . . As we move forward we must take care that our responses to commercial realities do not dominate the core educational, research, and innovative clinical practice missions of our school. . . . In our vision for the 21st century we should continue to be recognized for our extraordinary ability to make fundamental discoveries in biology and biomedical sciences. . . . We should continue to create unparalleled educational opportunities for our medical students, graduate students, fellows and house staff physicians, and to prepare them for leadership careers in medicine and biomedical research. . . . Ultimately we may find that we need a smaller more focused faculty.

The vision statement is very consistent with the place of Stanford's department of psychiatry within its medical school.

The residency program currently has 45 residents and is able to draw excellent candidates from around the country. Dr. Barr Taylor, the training director, projects that the program will likely downsize from 45 to 40 slots. He believes that the program will be organized around education tracks, including primary care, clinical neuroscience, and so forth. Drs. Schatzberg and Taylor were in substantial agreement on the five most critical skills for psychiatrists of the future—albeit with slight difference in emphasis (Schatzberg: diagnosis and assessment, treatment planning, communication with patients and HMOs, pharmacotherapy, and focal psychotherapy. Taylor: pharmacotherapy, brief psychotherapies, evaluation and treatment of complex medical/psychiatric cases, ability to work in teams, and primary care management skills). Research and advanced fellowship training will continue to play important roles in the future of this department's graduate medical education programs.

Relationship With the Department of Veterans Affairs

Critical to the educational and research programs of the psychiatry department is the viability of the Palo Alto VA Hospital. I met with Dr. Richard Maaze, an anesthesiologist who spent 6 years as the medical director and who is now the chief of staff of the Palo Alto VA Hospital. Traditionally, the Veterans Administration had two independently managed hospitals in the area: Menlo Park (a psychiatric and long-term care facility) and Palo Alto, focusing on acute medical-surgical and psychiatric care. There were 50 psychiatrists between the two facilities; only 9 held faculty positions. Palo Alto had 15 psychiatrists and Menlo Park 26. The Menlo division was autonomous and run by a psychiatrist who was proud that there was no academic affiliation with Stanford. Dr. Maaze believes that there were serious quality problems at the Menlo Park facility, including an inpatient drug program having an average length of stay of 280 days. The psychiatry services have now been integrated under Dr. Ira Glick as acting director, although the service is actually run by Dr. Javaid Sheikh, a consultation-liaison and geriatric psychiatrist.

Dr. Maaze has had significant conflict with leadership of the psychiatry service at Palo Alto, resulting in the resignation of the chief of psychiatry and several lawsuits by disaffected faculty members. Dr. Maaze disavows any hostility to psychiatry as a discipline, indicating that the VA is involved in a massive movement away from inpatient to ambulatory primary care. Specialty clinics such as hypertension and diabetes are being closed as new primary care clinics emerge. This shift is having a profound effect on the department of internal medicine. It is of interest that the VA is exploring ways to integrate psychiatry and psychology into primary care teams—and is in fact considering having psychiatrists as heads of some of these teams. As Dr. Maaze noted, "we have alcoholics and schizophrenics who happen to have problems with hypertension and diabetes." The model is interesting because the director of residency training in psychiatry, Dr. Barr Taylor, is looking for models to train residents in psychiatry with an emphasis on primary care. He had been unaware of the efforts at the VA.

The VA is also in the midst of activating a nonprofit corporation to receive grants that could deprive Stanford of significant indirect cost benefits. Dr. Maaze indicated that the faculty in psychiatry at the VA will continue to be strongly research oriented. No reduction below 50 psychiatrists for the two facilities was planned, and there was a hope that there would be up to 20 faculty among the 50 psychiatrists. Dr. Maaze envisions academic leadership for separate programs in inpatient, outpatient, consultation, addiction, geriatrics, and PTSD services.

Research Programs

As described earlier, the department derives most of its income from research grants (industry and government) and gifts and endowment tied to research programs. The department receives $1.1 million per year in pharmaceutical company support across 19 projects (9 of which carry Dr. Schatzberg as principal investigator). These clinical trials are linked to the department's growing reputation for clinical excellence. The department's substantial support from NIH is also tied heavily to high-quality clinical investigation on dementia, sleep disorders, psycho-social aspects of breast cancer survival, alcoholism, eating disorders, and stress.

In the past, the department had a large amount of grant support for molecular and human genetics of autism, as well as primate studies, and a coordinated program of clinical and neuroscience research. These pro-grams no longer exist, with the retirement of Dr. Seymour Levine, the premature death of Dr. Roland Ciaranello, and the departure of Dr. Jack Barchas and his colleagues. At this juncture, there are vacancies in the leadership of the Pritzker Lab, the division of child psychiatry, and the Goldstein Professorship in Addiction Medicine. Moreover, a major part of the current research portfolio is directed by individuals who may be close to retirement or are currently in a conflict situation at the VA. The child psychiatry recruitment is somewhat contingent on decisions at the children's hospital and the department of pediatrics. The high cost of clinical research space in the new psychiatry building compro-mises the department's financial situation. The grant support from in-dustry, in particular, does not include the type of money that could begin to help the department cover its space costs.

The bottom line is that it will be increasingly difficult for the de-partment to maintain its edge in research without substantial relief from its clinical delivery overhead costs, as well as strong support for current recruitment and planning for the retirement or relocation of key faculty in a number of areas.

Summary

The department of psychiatry at Stanford has a successful track record as a very strong research department in a school that highly values research. Its graduate medical education and undergraduate medical school teaching programs emphasize cutting-edge clinical and basic science. With the recruitment of the current chair, efforts were made to increase the department's involvement in clinical activities. The hospital reconfigured inpatient space for two units, and a new building was constructed for outpatient, PHP, clinical research, and educational purposes. This building, which replaced a prefabricated structure that was totally inadequate, has increased the apparent cost structure of the department within the new SHS. The latter has not really managed to transform the faculty practice into a multispecialty group, and it has certainly failed to address the unique management requirements of psychiatry (as primary care).

If some of the proposed arrangements with Kaiser and UCSF go through, the place of psychiatry at Stanford will certainly go through a significant change (e.g., location of beds). The department needs to recruit for a number of endowed professorships to replace faculty who have died, retired, or moved to other schools. Some of the most productive programs (e.g., the sleep disorders program and the behavioral medicine program) are uniquely tied to senior faculty members who are either close to requirement or based at the VA in a conflict-laden situation. Ultimately, if the department is to maintain its edge in research, it will need to be freed from the high costs of its clinical programs and the university will need to identify ways to foster recruitment of new faculty.

Index

*Page numbers in **boldface** type refer to tables or figures.*